Lessons in B

in B

to Enhance Your

and Joy of Living

breath
taking

Heal Faster

Relax Easier

Perform Better

LORIN ROCHE, Ph.D.

Notice

This book is intended as a reference volume only, not as a medical manual. The information given here is designed to help you make informed decisions about your health. It is not intended as a substitute for any treatment that may have been prescribed by your doctor. If you suspect that you have a medical problem, we urge you to seek competent medical help.

Epigraph by Marcel Proust from "The Captive," *Remembrance of Things Past* (vol. III). English translation by C. K. Scott-Moncrieff, Terence Kilmartin, and Andreas Mayor. New York: Random House, 1981.

Printed in the United States of America
Rodale Inc. makes every effort to use acid-free ∞, recycled paper ♻.

Cover and Interior Designer: Susan P. Eugster

Library of Congress Cataloging-in-Publication Data

Roche, Lorin.
    Breath taking : lessons in breathing / Lorin Roche.
        p.   cm.
    ISBN 1–57954–423–1
    1. Breathing exercises.   2. Respiration.   I. Title.
    RA782 .R634   2001
613'.192—dc21   2001001796

Distributed to the book trade by St. Martin's Press

2   4   6   8   10   9   7   5   3   1   paperback

Visit us on the Web at www.rodalestore.com, or call us toll-free at (800) 848-4735.

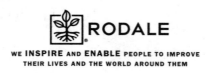

RODALE

WE **INSPIRE** AND **ENABLE** PEOPLE TO IMPROVE
THEIR LIVES AND THE WORLD AROUND THEM

*To the God
who breathes in me
and in all beings,*

*To the God
who breathes forth universes,
adoration.*

The only true voyage of discovery, the only really rejuvenating experience, would be not to visit strange lands but to possess other eyes, to see the universe through the eyes of another, of a hundred others, to see the hundred universes that each of them sees, that each of them is. . .

Le seul véritable voyage, le seul bain de Jouvence, ce ne serait pas d'aller vers de nouveaux paysages, mais d'avoir d'autres yeux, de voir l'univers avec les yeux d'un autre, de cent autres, de voir les cent univers que chacun d'eux voit [. . .]

MARCEL PROUST

CONTENTS

PREFACE

*T*his is a little book on how to fall in love with breath. It is an invitation to explore a world that is always there, a simple pleasure that's right under your nose, waiting for you. Learning to savor the rhythmic flow of the breath is a way to bring more joy into your life, enhance your sensuality, and be at ease in yourself and with others. Even the most basic and easy breath techniques can significantly help your health and your ability to perform well under pressure.

You can learn about breath by taking delight in your everyday activities: smelling your morning cup of coffee or tea, taking an extra minute to inhale the aroma of your food, relaxing into an easy breath rhythm for 30 seconds before walking out the door on your way to work, and witnessing the way that emotions change the texture of your breath as you go about your day. That's what this book is about.

The sensory quality of breath is infinitely nuanced. The exercises in the book lead into the process of exploring the way each of your many senses, instincts, and emotions shapes and flavors the way you experience a breath. Breath is lover, healer, chef, angel, spirit, radar, information agency, and massage therapist. Breath is a gift from God, and to gratefully accept that gift is a means of prayer. *Breath Taking* is written in such a way that you can explore and discover those ways of being with breath you truly love. One thing that listening to athletes, meditators, yogis, singers, dancers, actors, and other students of breath for the past 32 years has taught me: Everyone is different in the approach to and experience of breath. It is the most central, and usually the most neglected element, of any approach to performance, self-help, or therapy. You can explore *your* approach to breath and discover your favorite ways to play with it. It takes engagement and courage to find your own way, as opposed to just doing standardized exercises. But you are more likely to find techniques that work for you and that you will want to keep doing.

If you are taking a class or getting one-on-one coaching, so much of the pacing is dictated from outside. But breath is the last thing you want to give over to an outside authority. So go ahead, dare to be intimate with your breath; play with these explorations and enrich the life of your senses. You are already breathing anyway, even as you read these words. Enjoying the flow of the life-giving air is something you can do right now, and always, to deepen your experience of life.

INTRODUCTION
The Joy of Breathing

*T*here are moments when we stop taking life for granted and inhale deeply of the beauty that is around us. A cleansing breath drawn at glorious dawn; savoring the bouquet of a glass of fine wine before dinner; or, nestled in a lover's arms, surrendering to his or her smell—at such moments, you take life deeply into yourself and are intimate with something great. In the time it takes to breathe in and breathe out, you touch life and are touched by life intensely.

Miracles happen if you continue this appreciative awareness beyond the 3 to 4 seconds that such a moment usually lasts. To spend even 15 seconds in the same state, or 60 seconds, seems like a lifetime. And it can transform you.

Breath is a gift from God, a gift from the oceans and forests, from the universe. Breathing is, in fact, a relationship you are having with the natural world—a physical exchange with the sea of air surrounding the Earth. When you cultivate this relationship by attuning yourself to it, you are developing a gift that can bring you a lifetime of joy.

We can be interested in breath taking, fascinated by it, in the same way we are charmed by food, enchanted by sex, amazed by music. Most of the skill of aware breathing is in finding your pleasure circuits, those sensory pathways that light up when you breathe. Work at this; make a conscious effort to engage in your favorite activities with extra gusto and attentiveness. The more you link your adventures in breath to what you love—whether it is food, sleep, kids, horses, dancing, sex, or music—the better.

In my life, and in this book, I am greatly inspired by yoga in all its forms. I draw on it deeply. But I will not be using yoga terminology or imitating its methods. These are explorations you can do on your own, in the midst of your everyday life, so that you can develop your own yoga—what works for you to develop harmony among body, mind, and spirit.

Yoga is a Sanskrit word meaning "union," or joining together. The discipline of yoga is concerned with joining together all the elements of human life into one seamless, harmonious whole. The word is derived from an ancient Indo-European root, *yeug,* which occurs in English in the form of yoke, jugular, conjugate, subjugate, conjugal, enjoin, injunction, juxtapose, and syzygy.

The yoga tradition of India is astounding in that for several thousands of years, its followers have made a dedicated effort to notice and record every possible breathing technique and have accumulated a vast repertory of methods. They have cherished each insight into breath and formulated it into a short pithy statement, or sutra, so that it can be memorized and passed on from generation to generation.

Yoga techniques have been developed for every human activity. There is the yoga of work, the yoga of war, the yoga of eating, the yoga of meditation, the yoga of sex, the yoga of devotion to God, and thousands more. There is more to yoga than can be explored in one human lifetime, or even a hundred, and there is more variety than any one human being can comprehend.

There is, however, one overall impression of yoga that predominates in the popular mind: that of the reclusive yogi, celibate, poor, living apart from society in a cave or ashram on a mountainside. There is a lot of truth to this archetype, and indeed yogi monks have done much great exploration. Their work has been so powerful that their approach—denying life, denying sexuality, and in general doing the things that monks are supposed to do—permeates all of yoga. In other words, sub-jugation has been emphasized over conjugation.

As a meditation instructor, the approach I favor is to help people focus on becoming intimate with their own breath. When people tune in to their unique ebb and flow, they either invent the techniques they need to stay focused, or they are in-stinctively drawn to those that already exist and that naturally speak to them. This method of learning about breath may or may not be slower, but it's definitely more gentle than at-tempting to forcefully discipline your respiration.

The best things in life really are free. And if you are breathing easily while doing them, then they are even better. As you move through this mystery called life, you are often smitten with dif-ferent cravings: you want relief, stimulation, good food, com-panionship, a real vacation, and much more. It seems as if you would have to spend a lot of time or a lot of money to get these things. Maybe so. But first, explore what is right here, free for the taking, ready to enhance your health and your life right now.

For millennia, people all over the world have found breathing to be invaluable for inspiring and healing. This is the message from all the ancient traditions, from Buddhism and the Sufis to Zen and the Vipassana monks with their beautiful walking med-itations. Even today, singers and athletes testify that they can do what they do because they are centered in breath.

Breath is everyone's birthright. Its secrets are out in the open, under your nose, and inside you. I am convinced that the more people who know the secrets of conscious breath taking, the better.

So take a d e e p breath
— and let's begin.

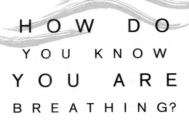

HOW DO
YOU KNOW
YOU ARE
BREATHING?

*B*reathing is by nature an intimate act. Atoms of oxygen and nitrogen that have been breathed by other beings on Earth for millions of years come into our bodies, are absorbed by our bodies, and are borne by blood throughout our bodies to permeate every cell. So we are already intimate with breath, and vice versa. And as with any intimate relationship, issues arise that must be dealt with: fear of intimacy, control issues, dominance, coordination, synchronization, and more.

It helps to be grateful, to cultivate gratitude. If we truly appreciate breath, something wonderful is added. If we spy on ourselves, on how we breathe, and make ourselves uncomfortable by being critical—which is, unfortunately, easy to do—then something is taken away: the feeling of freedom, of breathing easily. So let's approach this business of being breath-conscious in a positive way. After all, an intimate relationship should be enjoyable, even if what that means exactly is unique to you.

To start, if we were together I would ask *you* to tell *me* about breath. I believe there is little need for teachers to tell people things if they know what questions to ask. If someone came to me and said, "Lorin, tell me about breath," I would ask, "What makes you think there is such a thing? How do you know, by direct experience, that there is a process called breathing?"

This is not a trick. You have your own way of being intimate with breath, which is different from anyone who has ever lived. It is shaped by your favorite sensations and by your ability to love. It is limited by your fears, which are based on negative experiences in the past. We can safely assume that you are breathing as you read this, but how do you actually *know*? What informs you?

Become Intimate with Breath

Take a minute to entertain this question: *How do I know I am breathing right now?* Just wonder within yourself. You might want to rest your eyes on this page somewhere, or look at the horizon, or close your eyes completely. You can do this standing, sitting, or lying down. Just don't do it while driving or operating heavy machinery.

After pondering this question for five breaths or so, check

how you feel. Do you want to continue? If so, close your eyes and pay attention for 10 to 15 additional breaths.

When you finally open your eyes or focus again, think about what you experienced. If you say to yourself, *I could feel myself breathing*, exactly what did you feel? What kinds of details did you discern?

I could feel the air touching the inside of my nostrils as it flowed in.

I sensed the motion of my ribcage as it moved with the breath.

As I breathed in, my body expanded, and as I breathed out, I contracted.

I was conscious of the air sliding down the back of my throat.

The flow of breath is very soothing; I felt waves of calmness spreading through my body.

When I breathe out, I feel a great relief— I feel the fatigue washing away.

After considering this list of intimate experiences that others have had with breath, become aware once again of your own breath for another 10 inhalations.

Your experience will be different each time you do this exercise, even if you do it every day for the rest of your life. I always discover something new and surprising about breath. Part of this is because I am an explorer, and part of it is because my senses are so open to the world that I am able to perceive differences. What used to seem the "same" to me is now perceptibly different because I have more data.

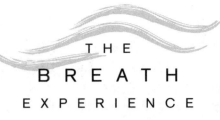

THE
BREATH
EXPERIENCE

*W*hen you take a conscious breath, you may experience any number of sensations.

Immediate relief	Sleepiness
Boredom	A sense of being at ease
Muscular relaxation	A flood of thoughts
Nothing much	Excitement and energy

There is no way of knowing for sure what your breath experience will be like because the interplay between the dimensions of breath—metabolism, information, and emotion—is infinitely complex. What you or I experience in any given moment of breath awareness is actually a side effect of what the body is doing as it balances its energies, heals itself, assesses the environment, acts on its instincts, and mobilizes to meet challenges from without and within.

There are two major aspects to the practice of breath awareness. The first is learning how to pay attention, which itself has
two parts: learning to ride the rhythms of awareness, and dis-
covering your favorite sensual pathways. The second aspect,
oddly enough, is learning how to handle relaxation. When you
relax, you come down off the stress response and you feel the
pain underneath—the pain of tensed muscles along with fatigue. Your mind may be flooded with images of what made
you tense, and your body will feel the sensations of tension
once more before letting go.

The process is similar to the experience of sitting on your
foot and cutting off circulation. You don't feel anything at first,
but when you restore circulation by standing up, you feel the
pins and needles. Almost every exercise in this book has to do
with restoring or increasing circulation, and you will experience
various kinds of pangs as you explore the conscious breath.
Rarely will you encounter anything as intense as what happens
when you sit on your foot. Mostly, they will be relatively tiny
sensations, but be accepting of them because this is how relaxation happens.

Personally, I love the stress response, with its tingling surge
of instant energy throughout the body. It saved our ancestors
many times, and I am sure it has saved my life at least a few
times. But, like a powerful motor, you don't want to rev your
nervous system needlessly.

Whether you are dealing with your kids or competing in the
Olympics, having just the right amount of energy is critical. In
the martial arts, sports, singing, or speech making, the ability to
relax in action is highly valued because it helps you perform at
your best. Breath awareness teaches you how to modulate your
stress response directly so that you can control your levels of
excitement and relaxation in any situation.

The more your senses evolve, the more you will notice how each moment is slightly different from any other. Mostly, you will experience what relaxation feels like. These sensations of winding down do not mean that you have failed in breath awareness. Rather, when you are at ease, your body will systematically review every time you have been ill at ease, to fine-tune its responsiveness. The different parts of your body will talk to one another. This is what human nervous systems do; it is an adaptive trait, part of our survival mechanism. It speaks to the success of your breath experience if the noise of the different parts of your body and brain talking to one another sounds like a cocktail party.

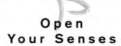

Open Your Senses

Arrange to sit somewhere comfortable where you won't be disturbed for a while. Sit upright in a chair with your back supported and your feet on the ground.

Sit for 1 minute with your eyes open and get used to just *being* there.

Notice that you are breathing, and open your senses to breath.

Find some aspect of breathing that is pleasant to you *right now*—the touch of air in your nostrils, down your throat, into your chest and belly. The rhythmic in-and-out of the breath, the massage of it, the quiet sounds. Focus on the sensation you like most and keep returning to this pleasure.

Your mind will always wander; the key is to be gentle in returning to the breath. In an easy and casual manner, keep bringing your attention back to the sensual experience of breathing.

When thoughts come, you will often become totally lost in them and forget that you are breathing. When you return from the thoughts, you will have a choice of what to pay attention to and again you can enjoy the breath.

You can practice this exercise for 1 minute, 3 minutes, 5 minutes, or even 20 minutes.

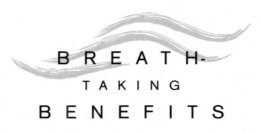

BREATH-
TAKING
BENEFITS

*P*aying attention to breath can enhance your life in a surprising number of ways.

- More enjoyment of work and play
- Enhanced performance when under pressure
- Greater ability to focus
- Sounder sleep; able to recover from fatigue more quickly
- Increased ability to establish and sustain intimate relationships with lovers, family, friends, animals
- Rapid recovery from stressful moments
- Feel time flowing in rhythm; you are relaxed and yet focused—"in the zone"
- Makes it easier to stop smoking or to minimize the habit
- Helps control weight by giving greater enjoyment from smaller portions, thus satisfying cravings
- More immediate access to intuition
- Added ease and grace as there is less unnecessary effort
- Able to energize yourself without relying on caffeine or stimulants
- Understand your own actions and motivations more quickly to correct destructive behavior

- Enjoy your food, music, sex, and playtime more because you are extra relaxed
- Rest more deeply than sleep
- Able to relax without alcohol or other drugs
- More patience; increases ability to listen to other people without interrupting

These goals are all fairly simple to accomplish; every day, people all over the world use breath to these ends. As part of their regular training, the following professionals receive instruction in breath awareness: athletes, policemen, physicians, sharpshooters, shamans, paramedics, executives, massage therapists, ministers, singers, actors, trance mediums, and scuba divers, to name just a few. You do not need to be in special training to practice breath awareness, however; you can elevate mundane tasks just by noticing how you breathe.

In essence I am saying *Take time to smell the roses.* In addition to the simple pleasures you'll get from everyday life, you'll be converting anxiety into excitement. This is no incidental side effect. As you breathe more freely, anxiety is transformed into the gift of energy.

Personalize Your Breath Experience

Consider these highly personal breath experiences, then think of similar ways that you would like to use your breath.

- A thirtysomething woman loves the smell of food. For her, that's the primary enjoyment of food—you can eat only so much, but if you get into the smell, the potential for pleasure is endless. The woman taught herself to meditate by taking comfort in the flow of breath. She sits down and takes breath with the same gusto that she breathes in delicious food smells. She meditates this way almost every day for a half-hour.

- A 45-year-old male singer, a Broadway star, has had more than 20 years of voice lessons. To him, breath is life—it gives him the ability to sing.

- Through studied breathing, an outdoorsman has developed his abilities as a tracker—a major feature of his life.

- A 55-year-old schoolteacher and mother has found that if she checks in with her breath throughout the day, she does not get as tired. And at the end of the workday, before dinner, she lies down and for 45 minutes does a complete scan of her body with the breath, which leaves her revived and refreshed for the rest of evening.

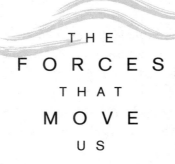

THE
FORCES
THAT
MOVE
US

*B*reath is extremely versatile, always adjusting itself to the needs of the moment. Notice how when you walk up stairs, your breathing rate increases. When you sit down, it slows because your muscles demand less oxygen at rest. When you are sleeping, oxygen consumption drops almost 10 percent. When you meditate, which you can do just by paying easy attention to the breath, your breathing rate slows down even more than it does in deep sleep. Being centered in your breath lets you slow yourself down or speed yourself up as needed.

When you breathe in, your body is refreshed with air.

You also receive information about your environment through smell, temperature, and humidity. Your emotional brain decides, on the basis of this information, how charged up to get, and your emotional muscles—around the ribs, the heart, and the belly—are massaged with each breath. Thus, the experiential dimensions of breath include metabolism, information, and emotional excitement.

Metabolism is the action of breath that feeds the fires of life. Every 4 to 5 seconds we breathe in several liters of air carrying oxygen that is then transported to the hundreds of billions of cells that make up the human body. The oxygen helps transform the food we eat into energy, motion, and heat. Indeed, our bodies are designed to need a continuous supply, and our cells start to die in minutes if starved of oxygen. Metabolism is maintained as we take in air, absorb oxygen, and excrete carbon dioxide into the atmosphere.

Information enters the body with every breath. Scents, temperature, and an incredible array of additional airborne data tells our brains what's happening in the environment. And as the air goes in and out of our bodies, the breath gives us knowledge of our inner conditions as well. Our breath lets us know what is going on inside and out.

Emotional excitement refers to the way we breathe to gear up for action or to transition into healing and resting states. Emotional tone varies widely, but one primary dimension is excitement—more or less, we are either calm or anxious in response to both outer and inner environments. Internally, breath is a continual massage of the heart, ribcage, and belly, and we use the rhythm to tune ourselves up for the activity we are about to engage in.

Breathing addresses all three of these dimensions whether we are conscious of it or not. Every breath you take is precisely modulated to meet your bodily needs and at the same time provides the environmental information necessary to inform your emotional response.

Breath is designed to be primarily an unconscious activity in human beings, but when we become attentively engaged with breath, we add a fourth dimension: consciousness.

Notice the Nose, Lips, and Mouth

The simple secret of this breath technique is to explore your breath as the most exquisite and satisfying type of touch.

Sit or lie down and pay attention to the sensations of touch created by the flowing air.

Breathe through your nose. When the breath enters your body, it touches first the skin around your nostrils. Just inside the nose are mucous membranes and many little nose hairs. Hair follicles are very sensitive to light touch.

Just by feeling, can you tell if you are breathing more through your right or your left nostril?

Breathe through your mouth. How delicately does a breath touch your lips if you open your mouth slightly as you breathe in? Take a few moments to savor the sensations of light touch, wetness, dryness, and the hot-and-cold differences in temperature as the breath flows over your lips and tongue and down the back of your throat.

Exhale through your mouth. Feel the breath flow through your lips, inside your mouth, over your tongue.

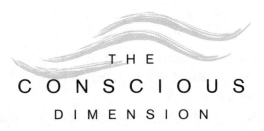

THE
CONSCIOUS
DIMENSION

*W*hen we engage with breath, we become aware that it is many things in one. To breathe in is to begin again. The incoming air swirls though the lungs and delivers oxygen to the blood. To breathe out is to be cleansed of the old air, the old thoughts and feelings.

Breathing is essential for life, although we take it completely for granted because we are supposed to; it's just too important for our conscious minds to manage. When you consider breath deliberately and respectfully, you add another dimension to the process, and a subtle magic happens. Breath is always helping us, keeping us alive, and adapting us to our environment. When we notice this, we become aware of the rhythm of life.

All the ancient philosophies revered breath and recommended developing an awareness of it. Breath *is* life—it is the ongoing gift of spirit. The Armenian spiritualist George Ivanovich Gurdjieff (1872-1949) said that breath is our primary food. In yoga it is called prana, and in the Chinese traditions, it is chi. Breath awareness is a component of all types of contemporary therapy: talk therapy, massage therapy, body therapy, hypnosis, postural work. Undoubtedly, there is more to breath than just air.

To be clear, consciousness does not mean control. Control can be a side effect, but if you go for control, you get mostly . . . control. Consciousness does not mean interfering with what is natural. If you are respectful, you realize that you are dropping in on a 400-million-year-old party that has been going on rhythmically without your awareness.

The first humans to become conscious of breath were probably hunters who mimicked the breathing patterns of their prey; mothers who discovered that they could soothe their babies by first matching their breathing and then slowing down; and lovers who learned to breathe together as part of the mating dance. Today, breath awareness is a popular technique to improve performance and add quality to our lives. You can see it at work in the Olympic diver who pauses on the board, visualizes her routine, takes a deep breath, then executes a beautiful dive. At the moment of truth, the breath becomes conscious.

Take 10
Conscious Breaths

Right now, if you have time, take 10 to 12 conscious breaths. That means you pay attention in some way, in your own way, as you breathe for the next minute or so.

Here are some variations to play with.

- Let your exhalations be slow—perhaps a deep inhale and a long, slow exhale.

- Depending on your mood and your physiological need, you might find yourself wanting to breathe rapidly. If so, give in to that impulse. Breathe rapidly in and out through your nose, panting as if you were running.

- Sigh as you breathe out. First, sigh as you would spontaneously. Notice the way you do it. Then slow the movement down slightly, giving yourself more time for the sigh. Do this at least six times.

- Take deep inhalations; on the exhales, shape your lips to make a sound—it could be any sound, perhaps a whooshing kind of a sound, or a *hu-u-u-u-u-u-u-u*. Notice the feeling throughout your body as you do so.

Take 10 conscious breaths anytime you feel like you want a little break—it takes less than a minute to get refreshed. In fact, it is good practice to do it every day because in a sense, all breath awareness work, all meditation, and all yoga is built on such a simple way of being with yourself.

If you want to explore conscious breath a bit more, get a pen and consider the question *What makes me want to breathe deeply?* Make a list of everything that comes to mind, and then explore them one at a time. Either in your outer life or in your imagination, visit those experiences that make you want to breathe deeply and take 10 conscious breaths to memorize the feeling.

Conjure up memories of activities that you really delight in. What, for example, is the best smell you can remember? Take a moment to cherish it right now. What is the most beautiful sight you have ever seen? It could be seeing a friend after a long absence, beholding a mountain, a loved pet running toward you, a thriving garden, or Michelangelo's Pietà. Or think of the most beautiful music you have ever heard, or the best caress you have ever received. Notice what happens to your breathing when you are imagining such things.

In the course of your life, you've experienced many of these moments. Now take a deep, satisfying breath and savor them. Get used to how close and accessible this quiet, good feeling is; it's available to you anytime. Thinking of things that make you want to breathe freely is a simple and wonderful way to get more pleasure from life.

Although this seems like a simple exercise, it is not trivial. For decades cigarette companies have been exploiting this technique by showing people smoking in scenes of great beauty and obviously fresh air. It was a brilliant marketing move to commercialize the human instinct to take a deep breath. Steal the impulse back and own it for yourself.

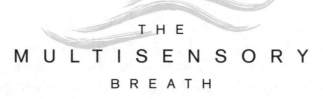

MULTISENSORY

BREATH

*W*e can enjoy the breath in an infinite variety of ways

and through all of our senses. Paying attention to any one

sense while being conscious of breath can be rewarding;

when we appreciate several of our senses at once, it gets

even more interesting.

First, there are the five physical senses we all know.

Hearing—The ability to decipher sound waves in the air

Sight—The ability to detect colors, shapes, textures, and motion within the visual range

Smell—The ability to detect odors in the air

Taste—The ability to detect salty, sweet, bitter, sour, or pungent substances on the tongue

Touch—The ability to detect light touch and deep touch through nerve endings on the skin

Then there are the other human senses, infinitely com-

plex and varied.

Balance—Orientation in gravity and acceleration; also called the vestibular sense

Barosensing—The ability to directly sense blood pressure

Chemosensing—The ability of blood vessels to signal the brain when carbon dioxide levels are too high

Joint position—The ability to know, without looking, the position of the joints relative to one another

Kinesthesia—The ability to sense movement anywhere in the body

Rhythm—The ability to detect the regular recurrence of a particular motion

Temperature—The ability to sense cold and heat relative to normal body temperature

This is not a complete list. Many more senses and feedback mechanisms operate within the human body, monitoring the incoming breath, the levels of oxygen and carbon dioxide in your bloodstream, and more. You have, for example, stretch receptors in your muscles to tell you when to yawn and stretch. With every intake of air, the temperature sensors in the mucous membranes of your nose tell you about the temperature and speed of the air, and the olfactory nerves tell you about the smell.

You have all these senses and many more, so use them. Take delight in them. Each sense is a marvelous world in itself as well as a gateway to the universe.

Bless Each Sense

Go through your senses—at the very least the five physical senses—and bless each one. Pet it, radiate gratitude to it, permeate that sense with your love of it for bringing you the world.

Attention blesses. It is a bit like gardening—planting, watering, removing the bugs, pruning. *When you pay attention to something, it blossoms.* Once you get this in your head, your whole path to self-awareness will be easier, safer, and much more fun. You'll be working *with* your inner nature, not against it.

It is usual for people to come to meditation or breath control at certain times in their lives: when they are lonely, grieving, or between commitments. It's those lonely nights at home when people explore. This phase typically lasts for a few months or years; then, they are off, married, with kids on the way, or something else. But the inner knowledge you develop in those dark times carries over, helps out. What you gain is never lost, even if you meditated only for that brief time and then never again. Here, now, at least once in your life, bless each and all of your senses.

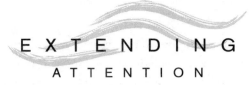

EXTENDING
ATTENTION

*W*hether you are poor, rich, or in between, you experience your life through your senses. Each of the senses allows you to experience breath—and the world—in a completely different way. As you pay attention to any of your senses, they become richer.

The senses are divine—a gift from God and the fruit of billions of years of fine-tuning by nature. They are the pathways through which we can enjoy our inner world and the outer world. When I talk about being conscious of breath, what I'm talking about first and foremost is being attentive to your senses as they tell you what is going on with your breathing.

People unnecessarily limit the amount of pleasure they

get from breathing. If you do not extend your attention into all the senses, when you *are* being mindful, your experience will tend to be monotonous and boring. The more you allow the richness of attention to guide you, the richer your breath experience will be.

People use the Internet to find jobs, companionship, education, shopping, news, and information on a dizzying array of topics and every hobby imaginable. It's employed in the service of every human instinct. You want your breath to do the same. Don't hit the ESCAPE button in life. Surf your senses. Let your attention move and flow. When it has finished checking things out, it will return renewed.

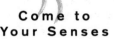

Come to Your Senses

For the space of 10 breaths, pay attention to the flow of breath with all the senses you can muster. Notice which pathways you come to naturally and which ones you have to work at. Let your attention orbit between the senses; then focus your attention simultaneously on all the senses. When you alternate senses, does the rhythm of your breath change? Which of the senses is most familiar to you?

Now I am aware of feeling the breath
touch the inside of my nose.

Now I am aware of smelling the freshness of the air.

Now I can hear the inhalation,
then the sigh of the exhalation.

Explore using a new sense, one you may never have paid attention to before. For example, notice your hunger for air. Can you sense the way your arteries continuously monitor the amount of oxygen in your blood and urge you to breathe again?

As I became aware of this hunger for breath,
I started yawning and sighing
and breathing deeply—it was almost
involuntary. I was craving air, more air.

I could hear the breath flowing in and out
with little sighing sounds: Ahhhhh.

When I breathe in cold air, it chills my nose,
and when I breathe out, the air is much
warmer, and I can see it, it makes steam.

All I could smell were the pine trees on that
mountain over there, very faintly but definitely there.

I had my eyes open, and with my peripheral
vision I could see my chest and belly
moving as I breathed in and out.

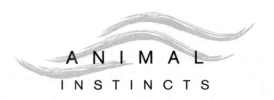

A N I M A L
I N S T I N C T S

*W*e have all heard the phrases "survival instinct" and "homing instinct." So what are instincts? They are the basic impulses of life. When we get hungry, we seek out food; when we get thirsty, we look for something to drink; when we need a place to live, we go hunting for one; when we feel the need for a mate, we start putting out signals that we are available. I like to think of instincts as the wise motions of life.

Instincts are the animal part of us, so be a healthy animal. Above all, do not hurt the instinctive energies inside you. For example, all mammals play, particularly when they are young. Little girls may play lawyer, doctor, mother, cook, or fireperson. Kittens play at attacking things—they practice the moves they will use later to catch mice. No one has to tell a kitten or a 4-year-old girl to play. No one should tell them not to. Instincts urge what's best for you.

If animals or humans hide from a predator, they instinctively quiet their breathing. The sounds of breathing are a dead giveaway, and all earth-bound mammals (as opposed to those who live in the sea) seem to know this: Once they stop running and find a place to hide, the body quiets their breath. So if your breathing feels restricted in any way, it may be because either you are afraid of something and are hiding, or you've been afraid of something for quite a while and breathing this way has become a habit.

When you are at rest or engaged in conscious breath taking, the brain instinctively sorts through priorities, unfinished tasks, and things you could have done better while checking in on survival strategies and attempting to choreograph the future. One moment you may feel as though you are gathering power, charging up; the next, resting, dozing off; getting excited, revving your motors; then, feeding quietly on breath.

This variety is what makes life interesting. Unless we specifically give ourselves freedom to range, there is a strong tendency to make up rules that shackle our instincts. In reality we are nurtured by all the forces of the universe—our eyes are nourished by light, our ears and bodies are informed by sound, our bones are fed by gravity. We can play, explore, feed, and rest in each sensory domain.

Do not submit to the traditions of yoga breathwork or the dominance of a traditional yoga teacher. That is imitative behavior, herd behavior. Rather, indulge your own instincts. If you let it, the wisdom of your body will guide you and make you more versatile. A childlike appreciation of the breath is necessary for this to happen. That is why I say that the techniques themselves are child's play and your approach to them should be also.

Stay curious. All creatures map their environments. Ants wander around looking for food, then race back to the nest and tell the others about it. Keep exploring.

Listen to Your Instincts

Examine your needs at this very moment: a vacation, more sleep, better food, comfort, a good laugh, a good cry, the rent money, or the sense that you are a good person capable of caring for those you love. These cravings are all deep and essential movements of life.

Right now, give some attention to those thoughts in the back of your brain and those sensations in your belly, chest, and shoulders. Give them permission to stand up and talk. Ask yourself this question and see what answers come up: *What needs, callings, yearnings, desires—instincts—are calling for my attention?*

Homing	Attending to offspring
Hunting and foraging	Exploring
Gathering and hoarding	Patrolling territory
Mating	Feeding
Nesting	Communicating

You may not think in these exact words, or in words at all. Perhaps you think in pictures—you may see a plate of food, a person to whom you are attracted or related, one of your children, a vacation poster, or your own front door. You might be feeling vague bodily sensations. It could take some unraveling to realize that the uncomfortable feeling in the pit of your stomach means that you feel threatened by the new person at work. Or, if you are feeling threatened in some more immediate or obvious way—you are late in paying a bill, you don't like the building that is going up across the street, or it suddenly dawns on you that you are 40—your protective instincts kick in and grab your attention more aggressively.

In any case, your instincts are constantly communicating your needs. When you rest, as in breath, there's a powwow of the instincts to determine how much you need to be aware of. As you do the exercises in this book, accommodate your primary instincts first and welcome whatever unexpected ones emerge. And remember that healing comes through balance— not just with rest, but in the balance of rest and exertion. In the same way, making contact with the inner self is not enough; balance is struck by sharing the self with the outer world.

A
CONSTELLATION
OF
INSTINCTS

*T*he more instincts you allow to inspire your conscious

attention, the more interesting your breathing will be. So

take some time now to consider which ones you love and

which ones you shy away from. Identify your favorite in-

stincts and scenarios. For example, if you like to go to

shopping malls, you are acting on your foraging and gath-

ering instincts. If you enjoy meeting friends there for

lunch, add socializing and feeding to your constellation of

instincts. If your favorite activity is to drink beer with

your friends and watch baseball on television, that is an

instinct for socializing as well as for group observation of

ritual combat. (There is an anthropological theory that

people invented civilization in order to have better access to beer: To make beer, you need not only a supply of hops but also clay pots in which to brew the beer. So somebody invented pottery. And to grow the hops you need a stable farm community. And there you go.)

When you enter your inner world through breath, the same constellation of instincts will be operating, although usually in a different sequence. As you breathe deeply, you are foraging for air, seeking to gather in an abundance of oxygen; if you breathe in with an awareness of those you love, you activate a very intimate bonding instinct.

You don't have to adapt instantly to your instincts in order to breathe with awareness, but whatever instincts you deny will shape your experience strongly. If you ignore your desire to play, for instance, and are always serious and working, that attitude will affect the techniques that you do—breathing, yoga, therapy, meditation, whatever.

As you become comfortable identifying your basic instincts, you will notice that your constellation rotates. You may be involved in acting on one instinct for a long time, then suddenly shift over into pure rest, delicious and satisfying. Then you might find your body flooded with erotic feelings as you start thinking about your mate. When you set yourself free to be with yourself, these are the kinds of things you will experience.

Breathe
with Each Instinct

Give yourself 1 to 3 minutes to settle down. When you are ready, breathe about five breaths with each of your instincts.

Recite each of the following sentences in your mind once or twice and then breathe with that mood. Pay special attention to the resonances that are evoked.

I am exploring the process of breath.

I am playing with awareness of breathing.

I am nesting, making myself at home with myself.

*I am resting, which I know makes
me able to function better.*

*I am feeding on the air, which I need
every minute to stay alive.*

*I am hunting for information and techniques
that will help me survive and be happy.*

*I welcome the breath into my body
as a lover welcomes her beloved.*

Breathe as a hunter, a mother, a father, a cook, a child playing, and a lover nestling.

To take this exercise further, pay attention to the sensations in your throat, chest, belly, pelvis, and throughout your entire body.

STRESS

*W*henever you take a moment to feel your breath, one of the first things you will confront is the stress you are under. You will feel it in your muscles and nerves, and in the thoughts that clamor for your attention. It is ironic but true: You may undertake conscious breathing expecting to express the quiet ecstasy of *Ahhh, what a relief*... but instead find yourself exclaiming "Man, my shoulders hurt!"

These days there are no saber-toothed tigers stalking us, but there are many other predators in the world wanting to buy the land out from under us, raise our rents, downsize our companies, downsize the country, change the economy, devalue the money we have saved, make us move, or make us learn new jobs. In the course of a typical day you may feel any or all of the following: bullied, hurried, trapped or boxed in, fear of failure, fear of being abandoned, worry over whether you can protect your children, overwhelmed, underappreciated—in a word, stressed.

The stress response in humans is extremely swift. You can be sitting in your office chair in utter safety on a physical level, and if your boss comes in and tells you that in 10 minutes you have to speak in front of the entire company within a second, your heart will start to race, your glands will start secreting hormones to activate your body for physical combat, your digestion will stop, you will begin to perspire, and the flow of blood to your skin will diminish so that if you were cut, you wouldn't bleed as much. Growth is delayed, pleasure is delayed, and cell repair and healing are delayed. In short, normal life functions are more or less put on hold while we are engaged in the stress response.

The good news is that you can start to come down off the stress response almost as quickly.

Breathe with Stress

Everyone is different in terms of what stresses them—some people are afraid of snakes and others have them as pets; some people are terrified of public speaking and others love it; some people are afraid of roller coasters and some crave the excitement. I have been swimming the Malibu coastline for more than 40 years, and in all that time only a couple of people have been attacked by sharks. But still, every time I swim over a patch of dark water, such as you see over a reef, my pulse quickens and my chest tightens.

Everyone is different also in terms of what relaxes them. Explore the following ways to breathe with stress when you're not stressed, so that you'll be ready when you are.

Heavy Breathing. Take three deep breaths and exhale slowly with a whoosh or a sigh. This is a natural move; you can see people doing it unconsciously when they have been under stress. By doing it intentionally, you are signaling to your system that it can stop pushing the emergency alarm. In about 15 seconds you should begin to regain your poise.

The Lookout. Move both your head and your eyes left, right, up, and down. Let your body see that there are no actual "tigers" crouched nearby. Face forward again and hold your head still as you move just your eyes left, right, up, and down. Then take three deep breaths, exhaling slowly.

The Belly Breath. As you inhale, let your whole torso expand, especially your lower torso. Practice this at least once a week while sitting or lying down. Find your favorite rhythm—there will be a speed you love. Even a couple of deep and slow belly breaths can be like a glass of wine—really good wine.

Paper Tiger. When something that is not an immediate physical danger scares you, give it points. *Good one! You got me going there.* This quickly changes the context; you are no longer a victim, you are playing. Then congratulate your body on the speed with which it hit the adrenaline button.

Dog Breath. If something is making you mad, honor that anger. As you breathe out, make a "grrrrr" sound, like dogs do. (If you are in public, make the sound very quietly.) This lets your body know that you are aware of the threat. Don't try to make it go away, just breathe with it.

The Shoulder Lift. As you breathe in, lift your shoulders high, then slowly drop them as you breathe out. If you are in a safe place, do this over and over for a minute, with great leisure. Do this for at least 5 minutes each week.

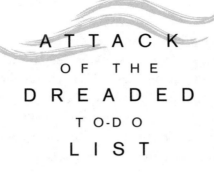

ATTACK

OF THE

DREADED

TO-DO

LIST

*W*hat sometimes happens when you first begin to relax in the breath is that you become aware of thoughts that you have been holding at bay. All of a sudden you remember the things you forgot to do or could have done better. Then you start remembering all the things you have way in the back of your brain but didn't have time to think of in the past week. This process is painful, like being bitten by fleas or besieged by tiny conscience elves with their sharp little pickaxes. Ouch.

You have opened the door from the top of your mind to the next level in. Now what?

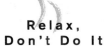

Relax,
Don't Do It

Say that you start doing one of the exercises in this book and within a few seconds you begin to feel relaxed. That sensation lasts for a moment but then you find yourself thinking of the many things you forgot to do today, yesterday, last week, and last year and feeling bad about them. There could be specific mental pictures, or it could be a vague sense of incompletion. What should you do?

Don't fight the feeling, give it space and time. Allow the process to engulf you. The human brain is built to know that there are many things that need doing, and it seeks to optimize the rhythm for accomplishing them. The brain is built to take advantage of any quiet time and use it for sorting through its to-do list.

This briefing/debriefing function of the brain is essential for peak performance. In situations where people really care about doing their best—in athletic competition and in the military, for example—there is a briefing before and a debriefing after. In debriefing, you review all the mistakes as well as the successes so that you learn how to improve your game.

The regret and embarrassment you feel during this process is a necessary part of learning. It's an aspect of your conscience: One of your instincts is saying, *Hey, you are neglecting your health/social life/money/housing/playtime/rest/work.* The intent is to help you bring yourself into balance. We are always neglecting some part of ourselves, some instinct, and that hurts. When we let this pain wash through us and we breathe with it, we stay connected to those neglected parts.

So accept every item on your mental to-do list and learn to breathe easily with them. Over time, the pain will pass and be replaced by pleasure, focus, or energy for action.

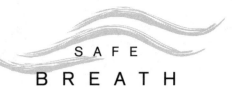

S A F E
B R E A T H

*T*here will be times in your breath taking when you encounter the feeling of being unsafe. It is possible that you are picking up on some real, imminent threat, yet it is more likely that you are remembering a time when you felt very unsafe. The feeling has come up now to be confronted and healed.

When you engage in breath awareness, you access massive amounts of data coming in through the senses, allowing you to make sounder judgment calls about how safe or unsafe you might be. In fact, we are usually very safe, even if we don't feel that way.

Sometimes you get to express your feelings, but at other times you have to put what you are feeling into the background and give another person the priority, such as

when raising kids, when listening to your mate, or when inter-
acting with coworkers. It may not be appropriate to throw
tantrums, break down, or spend a lot of time talking about how
you feel. So you build up a backlog.

The safer you feel, the more easily you will be able to release
your backlog of emotions. Paradoxically, most of this backlog is
about feeling unsafe—so when you finally do feel safe, you will
relax and feel unsafe. This effect is the bane of relaxation exercises. As you release the emotions, however, you will spontaneously start to breathe more easily.

The process is the same, whether you take 5 minutes to
breathe when you come home from work or whether you go on
vacation, go to a therapist, or go to a bar and have a drink with
a friend. One way or another, whatever feelings you have
trapped in your body will want to come to the surface of your
awareness and be spoken, acted on, felt, shared with others, and
released.

The basic principle is this: Pay attention to whatever emotions are calling you. As you breathe with them, they will get a
chance to resolve themselves.

Explore
Up and Down

Sit comfortably. On the inhale, let your head rock or tilt gently
back and upward. On the exhale, let the head fall forward slightly.
This is similar to the motion of sneezing, where the head moves
back on the *ah* and forward on the *choo*, except slow and easy.

The spine extends upward on the inhalation and curls down

a little on the exhalation. The chest rises and then sinks down and in. Get used to the different dimensions of motion. Continue this way for 5 minutes, your head moving just slightly back on the inhalation and then forward again on the exhalation.

Now on each inhale, stretch your spine ever upward so that you are sitting exceptionally erect. Make your head float up a little higher with each breath.

When you feel ready, project your spine right out of yourself. Let the energy coming off your tailbone extend down into the core of the Earth. Let the energy coming off your head reach up into the sky, as if your own personal sun is hovering above you, the sun of your soul, calling you upward.

At this point, this may seem like a mere exercise to you. If so, come back to it some day when you are feeling particularly in tune with yourself, some day when life, love, music, or another exploration elsewhere in this book has opened up your senses. Then it will be more than a mere exercise.

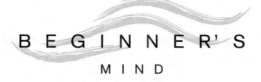

BEGINNER'S
MIND

$\mathcal{A}$ yoga teacher I know remarked that for the first 3

years she practiced yoga she had little interest in prana-

yama, the breath aspect, and that she felt uncomfortable

with the techniques. Then one day when her back hurt and

she couldn't do her ordinary moves, she discovered that

controlled breathing helped. Lying on her back, taking

ibuprofen, and humiliated, she found a new world open-

ing up to her. Each breath massaged her spine and rejuve-

nated her. She did not have to force anything; rather, she

finally surrendered to her natural instinct to breathe and

found herself letting go as never before in her adult life.

Prior to getting into yoga, this friend had gone through

a difficult divorce and had called upon her willpower to

help her forge a new life. Even after yoga had become a sacred refuge for her, however, she was unable to relax and truly let go. Striving, exercising her will, was what had saved her. Then that day, feeling how the breath was massaging her belly, her heart, the front of her spine, she relented. Now she teaches breath techniques enthusiastically, yet she knows from experience that it may take her students years to appreciate them fully.

Another time I was sitting with a wine merchant and I had him sniff the air, not so much for scent but just in appreciation—as the carrier for all the wonderful smells he had ever smelled. He instantly got what breath awareness is about and went into deep meditation, really enjoying himself.

One of the things students have taught me over the years is that there is no hierarchical organization to talent or intimacy with life. Beginners often know more than experts, and experts are often at their best when they come around to being beginners again.

Start with what you know. Everyone has something they do well, whether it is carpentry, keeping babies happy, or quickly sizing up a roomful of people. If you really know how to enjoy a freshly baked cookie, a glass of fine wine, or the scent of hay, then use that as a gateway into breath awareness.

Life tends to specialize us. Our senses become shaped by what we do. But humans are not ants. We were not born to be specialized. We ache to explore and see life afresh.

That possibility exists for you in every breath.

Caress
Yourself Inside

Lie down or sit down in any easy pose. For 1 to 5 minutes, exaggerate the inbreath and the outbreath. Give yourself a chance to really feel how moved your body is by the muscles of breathing. Feel how the organs in your belly are massaged.

Then for 5 minutes, rest and pay attention to breath as a loving caress, touching the inside of your torso, everywhere. There is nowhere the breath does not go; it is swirling inside your hipbones and breasts, and is delicately caressing the inside of your back and your heart. There are waves of breath gently billowing inside with infinite tenderness. Sit in a windy place, a breezy hillside, and as you breathe, experience breath as a massage.

Breath is continuous movement inside and out—the most powerful massage you could ever want.

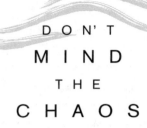

DON'T
MIND
THE
CHAOS

 s I got into a friend's car, she apologized for the mess. She works out of her car and had a cell phone, an appointment book, a bottle of water, two inspirational books, and a letter sitting on the passenger seat. In other words, she was living a life and had things to do. But still she was conditioned to say she was sorry: *Excuse me, I am busy living and don't have an extra house or car to use just for display.*

Over the years I have seen plenty of people approach meditation in a similar way. One part of their brain says to the other, *Excuse the chaos, please.*

When you start paying attention to breath, your mind

may seem totally cluttered, in complete chaos and disorder. But it is not. It is like the kitchen of a busy restaurant with dozens of people working together. Those stacks of dirty dishes are about to be attended to. Those boxes of zucchini are awaiting the prep cook. The people racing around shouting and joking are all very focused; it looks like chaos only if you have not learned to see the patterns. I have been learning and teaching meditation for most of my life—more than 30 years. Everyone thinks they are not worthy; that's the feeling we all have when approaching life's mysteries. Don't mistake humility for incompetence.

The biggest mistake you can make is thinking that you have to tidy up your mind. This is a huge waste of time. Just jump in and explore your breath and figure that within a few months you might understand what it is you're doing. The only thing that you need to worry about with regard to breathing is whether you are enjoying yourself.

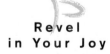

Revel
in Your Joy

Joy is a natural state of being, in contact with both nature and the self. There are many interesting textures of joy: exuberance, enthusiasm, and a kind of awe that existence exists at all.

To prepare for this exercise, you may want to listen to your favorite music or go to your favorite place. Alternatively, take a moment to recall three memories that bring you joy.

Inhale with a feeling of celebration. Drink in the air as if it were champagne—a ritual substance. Drink in the air as a toast to life. *I feel excited when I am aware of breathing, like there is so much life to be lived.* As you exhale, rest in the quiet feeling of joy.

Explore the natural movement of raising your arms in joy. Let your arms sweep upward and outward, expanding to welcome joy. Do this movement again and again, both quickly and slowly.

Inhale as you sweep the arms up; exhale as you bring them down. Reach, reach, and lift your face to the sky.

Open your arms as if you are about to embrace a long-lost friend. Then make the giving motion—touch your hands to your chest on the inbreath, and on the outbreath swing your arms wide, spreading joy to the world.

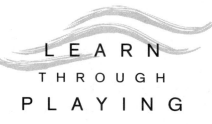

LEARN
THROUGH
PLAYING

*M*ammals learn their most important lessons through lighthearted play. This is why I disagree with breathing teachers who say that you must vigilantly watch for your mind to wander and then fiercely bring it back to what is important—the breath. This approach may be appropriate for monks living high in the mountains. Over time, they are able to make their mental soil so unwelcoming to desires that they lose the impulse to come down off their mountain and join the rest of us. But unless you are a recluse, there's no need to treat your thoughts like weeds.

In the approach that I recommend, you consciously cooperate with the impulses of life and bring the instincts into the breath by playing.

One of the most important things that teachers do is give permission. My students invent their own breath techniques. I believe that you learn from yourself, from your own body, from breath itself. So whether you are reading this book while sitting in a café or on your sofa or at the beach, the key is for you to give yourself permission to play. For many of us, this is no small matter.

Some of the explorations and meditations you may need to do only once before your body gets the hang of how to experience breath in that dimension. Other kinds of play you may want to return to again and again.

Explore
Left and Right

Put one of your fingers under your nose horizontally and feel the breath there. Can you tell if the left or right nostril is flowing more freely? If one nostril is completely blocked because of allergies or sinus trouble of some kind, wait until your nasal passages are clear to do this exercise.

If they are clear, flare your nostrils slightly on the inhale for a few breaths, just to put some attention there. If you like, sniff the air as you do so.

Become aware of your dominant hand—left or right. Don't move it yet, just become aware of it and your nose at the same time.

Let your hand float gently up to your nose. You will have to explore a bit to find the right position of the hands. What you want to do is to block alternate nostrils for one breath at a time. You don't have to block the nostrils completely; just use a light touch. On an exhale, lightly place your thumb under one nostril to block it and keep it there throughout the inhale. Then pause, switch nostrils, and exhale fully. Inhale fully, pause to switch nostrils again, then exhale. Continue for a few breaths.

This yoga move may seem awkward at first, but you just might be one of those people who come to love alternate nostril breathing. You won't know unless you explore it.

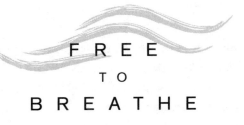

FREE
TO
BREATHE

*T*he body knows instinctively how to free up the breathing muscles. The problem is that you have learned to suppress this wisdom to get along in social circumstances.

For example, both shaking and saying "no" release fear. But if you are walking along and a big dog scares you, you might be hesitant to react in public. What you can do later is stand somewhere safe, stamp your foot, and shout, "No!" You may actually tremble or shake and then find that your breathing is freed up.

Releasing anger also frees up your breath. The key is to express yourself without hurting anyone. Whenever you feel mad, try to quickly arrange in your mind a time and place where you can let it out by hitting a pillow, throwing rocks into a pond—any motion where your arms and your whole upper torso get to indulge in the actions of anger.

Yawning and stretching are other ways your body frees itself up, loosening the muscles involved in breathing and feeling. In polite society we suppress yawning, but in so doing we constrict the muscles involved. Yawning is a natural yoga. Just look at babies. Babies are free with their emotions and with their breath. They scream, cry, laugh, rage, tremble, and yawn with total abandon.

Stretch and Yawn

Stretching and yawning are instinctive yoga moves. You can learn a great deal by indulging your natural impulses to stretch and yawn and noticing what movements and breaths your body invents. Oddly, this urge is so repressed that even people who are into their bodies often have never explored it. Think of it: A willing student will leave her home to drive to a yoga class that costs $15 an hour, yet she won't make the effort to learn from the spontaneous motions of her own body.

Right now give yourself permission to stretch and yawn, even if there are other people around. Get the ball rolling and then let the yawning and stretching reflex take over. Do not hurry. If your mouth is open in a big yawn, stay there as long as you can, up to 2 minutes.

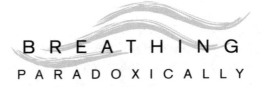

BREATHING
PARADOXICALLY

*P*ut one hand on your chest and one on your belly and notice their movement as you breathe. Does the air seem to flow down into your belly when you breathe in? Does your belly expand when you inhale, or does it tighten?

If you contract your belly when you breathe in, that's called paradoxical breathing. Health experts state the obvious when they point out that to get the fullest breath, you need to let your belly expand as you inhale. If you have been holding your belly in, relax and let it be filled by the breath.

It may feel strange to begin breathing in your belly if you have a habit of tightening your stomach to try to look thinner. But it is worthwhile to work through any awkwardness, for the future benefits to digestion and your ability to relax.

Take a
Belly Breath

Place one or both hands on your belly. Rest your hands there lightly and notice the motion of your belly as you breathe. Again, think of your favorite smells or things that you love, and notice what happens in your abdomen as you breathe. Continue this way for a dozen breaths or so—don't count them, just go for a minute.

Then place one hand on your belly and the other on your heart area, between your nipples. Rest your hands and notice what a comfort it is. There may be a very small, delicate good feeling in just having your hands in touch with these centers of breath. Do this for at least 3 minutes while either sitting comfortably or lying down.

DEEPER
THAN
SLEEP

*D*id you know that when you breathe with pleasure your body chemistry responds within seconds? Your blood pressure becomes lower, your heart rhythm stabilizes, and the volume of stress hormones in your blood decreases. In a single breath, you can begin to shift your mood from stressed to relaxed. After 30 years of clinical research, doctors now recognize that breathing in an even, full rhythm is one of the most effective antistress techniques.

A series of studies at Harvard Medical School found that by closing your eyes and enjoying your breath, which is a simple form of meditation, you tend to enter a state of rest that is deeper than sleep. Other studies have found that the levels of stress hormones in your blood will drop, and your immune system will be measurably strengthened.

Research indicates that during sleep, oxygen consumption decreases by about 8 percent over a period of several hours as the muscles relax and the body rests deeply. By contrast, when you do a simple meditation practice, the body enters a kind of conscious restfulness so deep that oxygen consumption drops by 12 to 17 percent in 3 to 5 minutes. This is a spontaneous side effect of the remarkable relaxation and rest meditation produces; it is not something you intentionally attempt.

Here is how: Sit comfortably for a minute or two, then close your eyes. Find an aspect of breath that you enjoy and pay attention to it in an easy manner without concentrating—just enjoy yourself. When your mind wanders, gently bring it back.

That's it—that's the procedure. It's called breath meditation, or breathing with pleasure, and anyone can do it. The capacity to slip into utter relaxation and rest at any moment is there in your body and nervous system, waiting to be used. It is a built-in instinct.

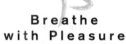

Breathe
with Pleasure

If you have a minute, take a breather. Give yourself permission, right now, to breathe easily. You don't have to adjust your posture, sit up straight, or change anything about yourself. Simply begin to breathe the way you do when you are experiencing pleasure. You might try imagining yourself in the following situations, taking one full breath while considering each item on the list.

- Smelling delicious aromas from the kitchen
- Walking along a favorite trail, street, or beach

- Looking at expansive vistas or fantastic weather displays

- Thinking of someone you love

- Participating in an exhilarating sport

- Being engrossed in a favorite hobby

- Dancing with passion

- Listening to a favorite song

- Arriving home from work or an extended trip

Select the one situation that seems most enjoyable at the moment and focus on how good it feels. Simply cherish the thought for a breath, then notice the way you are breathing. If another image or memory comes up, be with it also, then notice your breathing again.

If you don't have time now to practice this exercise, come back to it soon, for as simple as it seems, there is no end to what you can learn about yourself by being aware of breath and pleasure.

Human beings are constructed such that there is a great deal of pleasure to be experienced in the actions of breathing. This pleasure serves to root you in the reality of what life is, so that your sense of yourself and your decisions about how to live are based in a deep sense of connectedness to all life.

When you learn to monitor yourself in the present moment, you also have the opportunity to make course corrections in real time, rather than realizing later what you should have done. In other words, you are cultivating the ability to turn on a dime, to drop your expectations of what the situation should be and adapt quickly to what it actually is. When you take a conscious breath, you take in a great deal of information about your environment and your body updates its map of the world.

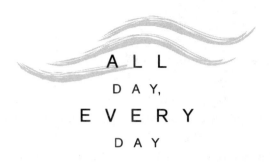

ALL
D A Y,
E V E R Y
D A Y

*T*his is how it could look if you played with breath as you moved through your day.

First of all, wake up into breath. Take a few deep breaths and stretch before getting out of bed. When you pour your morning drink—tea, juice, or coffee—inhale the aroma before downing it.

At midmorning, take a breathing break.

At lunch, pause for a moment to inhale the scent of the food before eating it.

When you get home from work, lie down for 10 minutes with your hand on your belly.

Before dinner, rest and be with the breath for 10 minutes.

Spending up to 40 minutes a day in breath exploration will reward you. You stand to get back more than you give, in either quality or quantity of time (fewer mistakes equals more net time). Being massaged by your own rhythm in this way will sometimes give you the feeling that everything outside you has slowed down and you now have an abundance of time.

Pause to Breathe on Each Threshold

One simple thing you can do as you move through your busy day is to shift speeds each time you go through a door. You can often shift your attention quite a bit in only a few seconds. You will know what the appropriate speed on the other side will be, or you can guess. You may need to speed up or, more likely, slow down, especially if you are arriving home at the end of the day.

As you get near your destination, become aware of your breathing. Feel any anxiety you have, which may show up as sensations in your belly, heart, or throat. Paying attention to the even flow of your breathing will soothe the anxieties and give them a chance to transform into positive energy. Anxiety is usually a sign that your body is storing nervous energy in case you have to fight or run away from a troubling situation. When you focus your attention on the anxiety itself, you transform that negative energy into readiness and excitement.

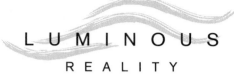

L U M I N O U S
R E A L I T Y

I grew up in the beach-town heaven of Southern California in the 1950s. Both of my parents were surfers, and I have spent much of my life in the ocean. When on land, I am usually within a few feet of the water, with the salt smell and ocean spray part of the very air I breathe. I sail, which involves reading the wind, and I surf, which means riding the waves the wind makes, yet for the longest time, I took breath for granted.

In 1968, while a freshman at the University of California, Irvine, that began to change. I became interested in meditation, partly in response to reading *Zen Flesh, Zen Bones* by Paul Reps. First published in 1957, this classic paperback introduced a generation of Americans to the concepts of Zen Buddhism. In the chapter on centering, there is a translation of one of the early teachings on meditation, the Bhairava Tantra, rendered by Reps as beautiful beatnik poetry.

This really intrigued me, and for a couple of years I explored this interest. I began meditating every day. I learned and then taught tai chi; I underwent a kind of deep-muscle bodywork called Rolfing, or Structural Integration; and I had a great many sessions in sensory-awareness techniques. My teachers kept directing my attention to the breath, but I wasn't really interested. Then one day, in the midst of a several-month-long movement-awareness workshop, it happened. It was like the sun rising on someone who had known only darkness. I began to experience breath as an elixir, something giving me life, and also as a friend—an intimate presence coming from the vastness.

Several years ago, I started work on my own version of the Bhairava Tantra, which was originally written in Sanskrit as far back as the second millennium B.C. Here is a passage on breath that illustrates why I call my translation *The Radiance Sutras.*

> *The way of experience begins with a breath*
> *such as the breath you are breathing now.*
>
> *Awakening into the luminous reality*
> *may dawn in the momentary throb*
> *between any two breaths.*
>
> *The breath flows in and just*
> *before it turns to flow out,*
> *there is a flash of pure joy—life is renewed.*
> *Awaken into that.*

I did awaken into this luminous reality, and breath awareness has stayed with me and developed over the years. As a part of my training as a meditation teacher, I sat in a totally dark room for 30 days. I experienced all the layers of human awareness, and all the terrors that anyone would when in complete isolation; but always there was the comforting pulsation of *something* keeping me company: my breath.

Breath awareness is not the domain of any one band of experts; it is by nature accessible to anyone and everyone. You can give over authority for many things, but no one else can take a breath for you. You must breathe every few seconds *on your own*, some 20,000 times a day. Like waves on a beach, the ocean of air flows in and flows out, again and again.

Awaken
to the Inner Fire

Light a candle and gaze at the flame for a minute. Notice how the flame pulsates and is itself breathing, drawing in oxygen from below and the sides, consuming the air, and giving off carbon dioxide above. Close your eyes and continue to see the flame pulsating in your mind's eye. Begin to breathe with the image of the flame.

Become aware that you are like a flame, drawing in air through your nose and mouth, into your lungs and bloodstream, and then to every cell. Each cell is a flame, combining sugar and oxygen to feed an ongoing fire. Imagine that a trillion tiny fires throughout your body are burning the oxygen. Rest for a moment in the awareness of flame, feeling it warm you and light you up from the inside.

Let your attention go back and forth between the little flame in your mind's eye and the multitude of flames that make up your body. In this, awaken to the radiance that you are. *Life is flame. I am flame.*

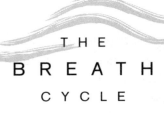

THE
BREATH
CYCLE

*C*onsider breathing as a four-part cycle: You breathe in; there is a phase where the breath turns from flowing in to flowing out; you breathe out; and there is a phase where the breath turns again, from out to in. Then the whole cycle repeats.

When you practice conscious breathing, give yourself over to the rhythm of the breath cycle. For a minute or two, simply notice the sensory pleasure of breathing in and out. Then slowly explore what aspect of the breath cycle you enjoy most. Your preference may change each time you do an exercise, or it may change from moment to moment. That's okay. It is the exploring, not the finding, that is relevant.

As you continue to pay attention to the breath cycle, a whole world of sensory experience gradually unfolds.

The silky sensation of air flowing
in and out of the body

The rhythm of the breath

The smell of the air: flowers nearby,
or someone cooking

The motion and undulation of the body
as the ribs expand into the inbreath
and contract with the outbreath

The quiet sound of the air flowing and whispering
through the same passages you use to sing and talk

The more senses you allow to come into play during the breath cycle, the more interesting and involving your breath taking will be.

Explore
Turning Motions

The breath does not just flow in and out. It also must make the transition from flowing out to flowing in and vice versa. These transitions can reveal to us the nature of change.

Pick a spot where you can pace back and forth. Walk one direction, turn, then walk back in the other direction, turn, then repeat. Do this for at least a few minutes, and as you do so, focus on the turning motion.

Now sit down and move your hands toward your mouth or heart area as you inhale, and then away from your body as you exhale. Pay special attention to the moment of transition, when your hands go from moving away from you to moving toward you, and again from moving toward you to moving away. Be aware of the sensations in your palms.

Move your palms in toward your chest, as if drawing in air. Move your palms outward, as if pushing out the old air. Continue this motion for 5 minutes.

Then rest your hands in your lap and pay attention to the flow of breath in the same way.

As the air flows in and out, pay attention to the rhythm: in, turn, out, turn, in, turn, out, turn. The turning point is neither stillness nor motion. It is stillness in motion, or sometimes motion in stillness.

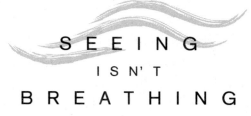

SEEING
ISN'T
BREATHING

*T*eachers of breath meditation often instruct their students to "Just watch your breath." This is an odd thing to ask, because of all your senses, the least helpful in appreciating breath is vision—ocular vision, anyway. (Your inner vision and your ability to visualize can add immensely to your appreciation of breath.)

When the air is clean, it is translucent, and light can travel for many miles. At night, we can see the sparkle of distant stars, photons that have traveled across the galaxy and through our atmosphere. So we don't usually see air, and we don't see our breath unless it's cold out and we can see the condensation as we exhale. (One of the appeals of smoking for me was seeing the exhalation.)

How else can you see breath? You can see the rise and fall of your belly and chest. This is significant because even though air is technically invisible, upon entering the body it becomes breath and thus visible in its effects. How magnificently complex.

Think of some of the vortices that you *can* see: the subtle undulation of steam rising from a boiling pot, or smoke swirling in the breeze. In the same way, as breath flows into and out of your body, it does not just go straight in and out but rather forms eddies, waves, and turbulence patterns that provide exquisite massage to your internal membranes.

Visualize
the Breath

If you could visualize the vitality that the air picks up as it blows through forests and mountain ranges and over oceans, what would you see? Would it be shimmering energy, liquid gold, microscopic dancing particles of light in the air? Explore this and find the images that you love.

If you were to visualize the outbreath carrying away the old air and feelings you want to be rid of, the old thoughts, how would you see that? Many people imagine it as an invisible smoke that carries away the used energies to be recycled.

When you find images you are attracted to, dwell with them on the inbreath and the outbreath. See every cell of your body being filled with vibrancy and life on the inbreath. And as you breathe out, see the outgoing air carrying away everything you no longer need as the carbon dioxide flows out.

This practice is as simple as child's play and yet it is something you can benefit from immeasurably over the course of a lifetime.

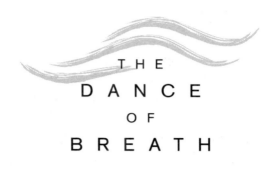

THE
DANCE
OF
BREATH

And take upon's the mystery of things,
As if we were God's spies . . .

—WILLIAM SHAKESPEARE, *KING LEAR*

*L*ife is an interplay of cosmic rhythms. Galaxies swirl, planets spin, and suns radiate and occasionally explode. The rotation of our Earth gives us night and day, summer, fall, winter, and spring. Plants and animals behave and breed according to the seasons.

We humans move in our own cycles. We work certain hours in a day, certain days in a week. We have daily routines: We read the morning paper or listen to gossip, check our e-mail, attend meetings, eat at favorite restaurants, and check in with friends. Breath is a continual motion through us, a tango in which oxygen atoms given off by oceans and plants travel toward us, pass into our bodies with the inhale, and then are blown back out, transformed, on the exhale. There are many levels of movement to be enjoyed.

For a vital process, breath is unusual in that it is both involuntary and voluntary. Breath goes on day and night whether we will it to or not, but we can also alter the rhythm if we want, or even, for a short time, hold the breath.

Breath has speed, motion, rhythm, and pauses, all of which differ in quality and quantity from person to person. What doesn't differ is the breathing cycle: inhale, turn out, exhale, turn in. If we breathe at an average rate of 16 times per minute, then each breath cycle lasts approximately 3.75 seconds. That's about a second and a half each for the inhale and the exhale, plus a mere fraction of a second for each turn of the breath. If someone is breathing relatively slowly, at say 12 breaths per minute, the breath cycles every 5 seconds. This is closer to where we want to be for conscious breathing.

Breath is part of every human movement, every action. Athletes, dancers, singers, and yogis know this. Notice the tempo of your breath the next time you are engaged in your favorite activity.

Rhythm is about the play of opposites: up and down, in and out, expand and contract, I and not-I. What I want you to realize is that you have your own rhythm. Dwelling in the involuntary motion of your breath is a kind of acceptance of yourself. You can lie still, release all control, and still be moved in a unique way by your own breath. You can also use breath to speed your pace up or slow it down. Let your breath remind you to move at your own rhythm.

Witness the Play
of Thoughts and Silence

For a minute or so, close your eyes and welcome the dance of your thoughts. By thoughts I mean bodily sensations as well as mental images. If you have ever tended animals, you know that when you show up, all of the animals come over and look at you and make their sounds, waiting to be fed. In the same way, your thoughts come to you to be fed attention and maybe petted a bit.

The visual content of your thoughts can appear as a series of stills or as quick, MTV-type flickering montages that mix moving images with fixed mental pictures. The audio portion of your inner conversations can mirror the way you are talking to yourself right now, take the form of a replay of something that someone once said to you, or sound like babbling background chatter or the words to a popular song.

You can even think with your muscles. If you sit in a chair and think about doing a favorite activity—dancing, hugging your children, swimming, walking through the shopping mall—your muscles might move just a tiny bit in response to the images. The same nerves you use to actually move are stimulated in imagination. This phenomenon can be measured by an instrument called an electromyograph, or EMG.

A MULTIDIMENSIONAL PATH TO THE SELF

*T*here are different pathways to breath awareness.

Breath is always in **motion**, creating a continual rhythm within you. Inside, you have sensors to detect this motion and instincts to keep it in balance. Motion always provides information, in this case about the inner world, and adaptation. Like the touch of your breath, the motion of your breath can calm you down or accelerate your metabolism according to the needs of the moment.

The **touch** of breath is nurturing—we feel fed by touch, we gain information by touch, and touch can stimulate or calm. Plus you can experience breath as one continual massage.

Even though there is not much of breath that you can see, **vision** is an important pathway. Human beings can learn simply by visualizing. We can rehearse new behaviors as well as understand what we are doing through inner vision and imagination.

Gusto allows us to appreciate the sensations of smell and taste. Like breath taking itself, smell is not just about drawing in the breath and exhaling it. Smell provides information about the environment and generates emotional connections. Smell also can heighten consciousness.

The song of breath, its **sound**, is food for both soul and body. When you listen to the song of breath, you realize that you can bathe in, drink, and eat sound. Breathing is the basis of speech, and by listening to the sounds themselves you can learn a lot, share information, or have a good time. The sound of the breath can be rousing or soporific.

Your **energy centers**, the places in the body where many nerves come together, are activated and informed by breath. These centers, which are found in the pelvis, belly, heart, head, and many other places in the body, are the loci of your delight, so get to know them.

Breathing with an awareness of **emotion** allows the energies of emotion to feed us. Rest is nurturing, excitement is nurturing. Breath informs us about our emotional responses to the world and gives us the means to support each emotional state. Emotions themselves are dependent upon our need to adapt and our energy stores.

Breath is intrinsically sacred, and to witness its comings and goings is regarded as a **prayer** in itself.

Every breath is a miniature **adventure**, one step into a new world on the quest to renew and refresh life. There are challenges and allies on the path to breathing freely.

Notice
Multidimensional Motion

Lie down, put a pillow under your knees, and place your hands on your belly. If your neck is tight, put a little pillow under your head. You could even drape a towel over your eyes to block out the light. Then notice and experience each of the following types of breathing motion.

Involuntary motion. Put your attention on the motion of your belly as you breathe; don't *do* anything. Let go of willpower and notice that the flow of breath continues without any doing on your part. This is a very simple observation, and you can get it in a few seconds. *Life moves with me and through me without any trying on my part. I can rest in myself and witness the dance of life.* If your breath is not effortless, if you have asthma, allergies, emphysema, or a cold, then notice the way your breath continues without your will.

Gentle motion. Move your body a small amount in sync with the breath. Just a tiny motion of the torso, suggested by the breath motion itself. Notice what it is like to cooperate with breath. It's like swinging on a swing, when all you have to do is lean into the swinging motion to keep the pendulum effect going. Feel for the moment in the motion when you can augment the act of breathing.

Deliberate motion. Make yourself breathe any way that occurs to you—deeply, rapidly, with no belly movement, or with belly movement. Just do it intentionally and with effort.

Each of these breathing motions uses your nerves and muscles in unique ways, and each is valuable in its own right. Learn to appreciate each, and learn to switch quickly from one mode to another.

There is a place for effort and intentional movement in breath exploration. Learn to notice when you are making an effort, when you are making just a slight effort, and when you are allowing the body to breathe by itself. Some people find that they always are making an effort, even when it is not necessary, because they are afraid they are doing it wrong. Thus, when they pay attention to anything, including breathing, they interfere with what is happening naturally. This is a subtle knot to untie because you can't try to not try. The way through this is to simply notice and honor each type of motion, whether it is involuntary and spontaneous or deliberate. You will find that you will learn to pay attention to natural motion and not interfere with it, just enjoy it.

When you are able to distinguish and engage in all the modes of effortlessness and effort, you will have developed a dexterity of breath that will serve you in life, work, and love.

GUSTO

*L*iving with gusto means really smelling and tasting life—taking delight in the taste of your own life, getting the juice out of it. Gusto is a way we approach food and drink, eating with zest and total enjoyment. Food is nourishment, but it's also sensual and can even be healing. Breath is a vital part of eating because smell is 80 percent of taste. So let's explore some ways to bring more gusto to the breath.

The sense of smell is the brain touching the air—smells go right to the brain. We may not be aware of it, but we smell the air with every inhale, and we inhale every 4 to 5 seconds, day and night. Our brains keep track of the incoming information and ring the alarm bells only if there is something apparently wrong.

Smell evokes sensations that go all the way into the belly, and when you smell something good, breathing is freed up spontaneously. The purpose of this chapter is to magnify the feeling of being nourished by breath: You can draw on it, even demand from it whatever qualities you need to feel nourished. This ability will encourage breath awareness and will give more texture to the breath techniques you do.

When we inhale, we inhale the world. Smell is the first sense that tells us it's okay to breathe because the air is breathable. The incoming oxygen feeds the fires of life—every cell in the body requires a constant fresh supply. So if you lack gusto, you are missing out on much of the vitality that is available just a breath away.

Explore Your Favorite Smells

Think about which smells make you feel excited, nurtured, spiritual, sexual, peaceful, restful. Now go seek them out and spend some time breathing with each.

While you are exploring, notice which smells incite you to breathe particularly deeply. What smells make you happy? You may have to hunt for them, or you may know them immediately. It may involve venturing out into the garden, or to the ocean, or into the kitchen: a fresh peach, a blade of grass, a leaf, some coffee beans, a drop of perfume on your wrist. Hunt for new smells. If you have already had the experience of sampling fragrances at the department store perfume counter, visit a shop that carries essential oils or the raw ingredients of perfumes.

Employ your other instincts. What smells make you feel playful? What smell is truly tantalizing to you, and how much of it can you tolerate?

Once you have thoroughly explored your own favorite smells, consider which smells stimulate your partner. Say your husband likes to tinker in the garage. Go out there sometime to visit him and get into all the smells: the wood, the glue, the oils, the gasoline, and the other odors that delight him so much. Without saying much about it, just enjoy these smells immensely.

Men, ask your woman to share her favorite smells with you. She will lead you into her secret world if you enter with respect. There may be places nearby where she pauses while walking to savor the smell of a tree, a bakery, or a lake. There may be an open vista where a breeze blows and the air just smells fresh. In the house, she may have stashes of vanilla and cinnamon. In the closet, she might delight in the smell of a leather jacket. Open your senses to enjoy whatever aromas she really likes. Ask her to put perfume on her body, rub against you and mark you with her scent, and then let her smell how it interacts with your skin. And at least once in your life, accompany a woman to a department store and spend an hour just inhaling the smell of the perfumes and learning what that is all about.

HUNGER

*H*unger can be a pleasant, even ecstatic, sensation. Anticipation, eagerness, and readiness are all part of the joy of eating. Physiologically, hunger is a sense; a whole array of sensors throughout your body tell you that it is time to get more fuel.

In many cultures, gathering before a meal is part of the ritual of everyday life. You smell the food being prepared as you sit and chat. Minute by minute you get hungrier and hungrier, salivating at the scents coming from the food as it cooks. This delightful torture gets the digestive juices going—you may have noticed that when you eat under such conditions, the food not only tastes better but also is digested more easily.

The so-called health food movement has done a lot to

destroy healthy appetites. There is so much conflicting information and fear about food. We get the sense that everything we eat
and drink is full of poison. Being exposed to this hype diminishes
the joy of living considerably, and is itself a kind of pollution—
information pollution. I have been around health food fanatics
for more than 30 years and I have to say that only a small per-
centage of people thrive on health food. In some places in California, you have to interview houseguests to find out if they: a)
are vegetarian, b) are vegetarian except for fish, c) are vegan, d)
will eat beef and chicken, e) eat only organic foods, or f) are any
combination of low-fat, no-salt, no-dairy, and free-range. (Even
so, your guests may have no problem eating the richest, most
lavish desserts possible, as long as the chocolate-truffle cake is
made with organic chocolate and cream.) This diet fanaticism is
a way people define themselves—like tattooing—but it is a huge
sacrifice of vitality. Even young, healthy people have become
afraid of their food and the water coming from their tap. By contrast, people who trust their instincts about what to eat and really
enjoy their food seem to be much healthier.

Honor Hunger

Put yourself in a situation where you feel hunger and you can
smell good food.

You could go into your kitchen and cook up something yourself. See if you can tell by smell alone when the vegetables are
almost done. Or go visit someone who loves to cook and ask
him to first tantalize you and then feed you. Or go to a restaurant and sit near the kitchen.

However or wherever you do it, inhale the delicious aromas for at least 10 minutes, all the while focusing on what's happening in your body. Where do you feel the hunger? What are the sensations? Enter into these sensations with your total awareness—it's an amazing experience, as powerful as a drug.

Increase your tolerance for hunger by practicing deep and slow breathing. You will tend to do this anyway if you are hungry, and it is a very healthy practice. Sometimes the things people do spontaneously are the best techniques of all. An excellent time to try this exercise is at a holiday dinner, when family and friends come together, sit at the table talking, and then wait, seemingly endlessly, while aromas waft from the stove.

Whenever you are in such a situation, whether at Thanksgiving or on a weeknight at the local diner, give thanks for your sense of smell. Give thanks for the air flowing in. Notice how the smell itself seems to feed you, to feed something deep inside you.

When you are gathered with other people waiting for a meal, many instincts are active at once and there is a kind of a melody to the proceedings. You may feel your body resting, sinking back into your seat, especially if you journeyed far. There is socializing, and updating one another on kinship issues as well as your map of the world. There will be laughter, perhaps singing, and general expressiveness. A good conversation over a meal is really a yoga of instincts, an event in which many different life impulses come together and are integrated. This is the experience you want to study, breathe with, memorize, so that you can give it to yourself even when you are eating out of a paper bag at work or alone in your apartment or home. If you can access this richness instinctively, you will also be better at giving it to others—and everyone hungers for something.

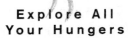

Explore All
Your Hungers

Hunger doesn't just pertain to the desire for food. Humans have many hungers. *I hunger for your touch, I am hungry for the light in Salzburg, I am hungry for good music, I am hungry for companionship.* We use the word *hunger* to refer to an appetite for life.

Breath awareness offers a very subtle way of dealing with your appetite for life. This exercise is very simple, but profound.

Identify any hunger that arises in you—for any of the qualities mentioned above, for spiritual experience, for travel, for adventure—and condense that sense of hunger into one descriptive word. Think that word as you breathe in.

Sweetness	Peace	Safety
Love	Adventure	Freedom
Delight	Companionship	Clarity
Fun	Solitude	Rest
Depth	Silence	Comfort

When you breathe in as if you are smelling a quality, you are feeding on that quality. Your body acts as if you are being nourished by that quality, and there is a profound sense of satisfaction. This is not an illusion—your body, nervous system, and awareness are the means by which you will get to where you are going in life. When you imbibe the quality of what you are craving by thinking of it on the inhale, you are breathing yourself one step closer to living your dream.

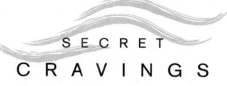

SECRET
CRAVINGS

*E*xplore your secret cravings—the tastes and smells toward which you are inevitably drawn and sometimes even seek out. Notice which smells you feel okay about saying "I love that" and which smells you like but have never told anyone. For example, I love the smell of WD-40 but have never told anyone. And I love, in a haunting, powerful way, the smell of fiberglass resin as detected from about 30 feet away when a surfboard is being made.

Whenever you can do so without harm, indulge your secret cravings through your sense of smell. You can get your fill of fattening foods without putting on weight or ingesting unhealthy cholesterol—buy the very best chocolate you can find and inhale the scent with gusto.

Smell is not a polite sense. When you really awaken to smell, you will have the experience of inhaling odors as if for the first time, and you may find that you love the smell of sweat. Your tastes may change, too. A food that you thought was your favorite may not be anymore. You probably used to like it, but if you were to taste it for the first time today, would you still?

Also, if you have been resisting a craving because you used to overindulge in some food, you may find that you can eat it now in moderation, or have lost your taste for it completely. When we resist a craving, we may lose contact with our sense and only *think* we crave something when actually our taste has moved on.

Our habits are sustained by inattentiveness. Perhaps once, long ago, we liked something and it became part of our routine. But when you awaken your senses, they bring you news every moment. By paying close attention, you will become more self-regulating, instinctive, and accepting of your cravings.

Cherish
Scents

Make yourself comfortable somewhere—on your sofa, in the garden, in a forest, by the beach, or in bed. Have one or more scents on hand, perhaps contrasting ones; anything you love the smell of and want to explore: different kinds of fruit, essential oils, leather, a cigar, flowers, or herbs.

While lying down or sitting, hold the scent near your nose and inhale its fragrance. Notice how your breathing changes as you cherish that smell. Then, if you are holding it near your nose, put your hand down and continue to be aware of breathing, enjoying the aftereffects of the smell.

Then hold the scent close to your nose again, but not as close. Again, notice what it feels like to breathe in a deep, cherishing breath.

Next, hold the fragrant item even farther from your nose, so you detect just a faint trace of the scent on the inbreath.

Now rest your hands in your lap, or if you are lying down, put everything aside, and simply enjoy breathing air. The air may have faint particles of scent, but there is something wonderful in plain old air itself.

Continue this way for several minutes. If you want to rest really deeply, you can continue for up to 20 minutes.

THE
SMOKING
SECTION

*I*f smoking weren't bad for you, it would be good for you.

Every hour or so, when you take a smoke break, you get
to lean back and take deep, yogalike breaths, doing a slow
exhale as you dramatically blow smoke into the air. Or
maybe you stand on the balcony with the other smokers
and gossip. In any case, the cigarette is a built-in timer;
you can be unaware of time for a moment and then in a
predictable 3 to 5 minutes, the cigarette goes out and your
break is over. Study after study has shown that people are
more productive, whether they are slinging bricks or paper
or electrons, if they take a short break every hour. If you
take the cigarette away and do the rest of the ritual, it be-

comes a breathing break. For 2 minutes or so, just breathe and enjoy the air as if it were an illicit pleasure.

Human beings have been around smoke for a long time, at least since fire was domesticated ages ago. After all, where there's fire, there's smoke. Think of our ancestors sitting around the fire all those long nights, struggling to invent language so they could tell stories and gossip instead of just waving their arms around. Think about how they might smell—smoky.

If you have ever been around a campfire, you know that at least half the time you are inhaling smoke. And if you are in a contained space such as a cave or a hut, the smoke gets thick. Fire was a friend for its warmth, for cooking, and for scaring away dangerous predators. The trail of smoke in the sky was a handy way of finding your way home after a long day of hunting and gathering. Smelling the smoke meant you were almost there. Smoking has deep, primal roots that have a stronger hold on us than nicotine.

When I ask smokers why they do it I get all kinds of interesting and unique responses.

- "I like the in-your-face attitude of smoking."

- "I hate it, and I know I'm addicted, but I do like having an excuse to go outside every hour and stand around. I think I'd go crazy or quit my job if I didn't do that."

- "I like the feeling of the smoke coming down and swirling around my heart. I can feel the smoke right there on the inside of my sternum [thumps chest]. That is where my heart is. I want to feel my heart touched."

- "It is a slightly dizzy sensation. I want to be taken, to be a little off-balance for a moment. It means I am wild inside."

One night I witnessed a scene that you could see almost any-where on Earth. I had stopped at a gas station, and while I was waiting to fill up I observed one of the attendants walk off the property a few feet and sit down on a curb in a relaxed pose. He took his pack out, looked at the flame as he lit a cigarette, and then tilted his head back and sighed. As I watched, he held the cigarette in his hand and sighed again, and at the end of the exhale he slumped a little and dropped his head down, letting go very deeply for a moment. Then he lifted his head and looked at the horizon, dreamily, through the smoke. For the moment, he shed the demeanor of a man who works the late shift in a gas station. He was himself for a moment. You could tell that in his mind he had every right to be sitting there doing what he was doing. He was sitting on a curb in a commercial street but he owned that spot for the moment. I don't know if it's because the cigarette break is sacred, if the smoke is an in-cense that propitiates some god, or because you buy the right to do breathing exercises when you pay to breathe smoke.

Another evening I was taking a stroll when suddenly I was seized by a strong craving for a smoke. So I did the following exercise, which has you explore your craving. I found that I wanted the feeling of my lungs being really full. I wanted sen-sation in my entire ribcage at the end of the inhale, and I wanted that extra-rich sensation of the smoke blowing over the back of the throat on the exhale. What I really didn't want was to start smoking again. So while walking along, I had to invent a little breath technique. I paid attention to the turn at the end of the inhale in a special way I had never noticed before, and as I was exhaling I brought my tongue up to feel the air going out. Then the craving was fulfilled.

About 20 minutes later I was walking back the same way and there were lots of people standing on the sidewalk outside of a restaurant smoking and having a good time. I was completely neutral. I enjoyed them and their banter without even a tiny blip of attraction for a cigarette or revulsion at the smell of the smoke.

Draw Breath
Instead

When you crave a cigarette, go into aware breathing. If you are walking, continue walking. If you are working, continue working, but have some awareness of the breathing going on.

If you gave up smoking, you can do the exercise to recover the good that was in your smoking habit. There is always something good in a habit, something positive that the body is doing. With aware breathing, you don't get into a struggle with the desire; rather, you experience the desire as a thing in itself. So when the craving hits you, give attention to it, so that the positive qualities underneath can emerge. If you still smoke, you can do the exercise and then smoke your cigarette.

1. As soon as you notice a desire to smoke, pay attention to your lips, your tongue, your throat, and finally your lungs.

2. Take three very slow breaths, noticing the way your ribs expand in all directions when you inhale. This is to relax you and open your senses. Then return to your lips, tongue, throat, and lungs, in that order, and note what sensations, feelings, or yearnings are there.

3. Ask yourself, *What am I craving?* Give the impulse or craving a chance to get stronger and clearer. We rarely do this, and this is the secret of the exercise.

4. Wonder to yourself, *How would my breath feel better if I* *were smoking?* Then notice what responses you get from your body. Remember that your body speaks in the language of sensations, not English. The sensations of desire may get stronger still, or they may change.

5. Then ask yourself, *Where am I craving?* The craving must be located somewhere inside your body. Try to pinpoint what part of your breathing system or body is saying it needs something.

6. Now find a way to give yourself that something through breath. What is good about the sensations you would have if you smoked a cigarette? Give it to yourself right now. You may have to invent a breathing technique that satisfies you.

DISGUST

One day I noticed a bad smell outside of my house. It got worse the next day. I sniffed around, and my nose told me that this was the smell of death. It was a hideous, alarming smell. We had thick ivy covering the fence, and a dead possum was rotting in the undergrowth. The smell said very clearly: Stay away—Nature is at work turning this possum into compost.

The opposite of gusto is disgust, and another function of smell is to inform us when things are rotten or toxic and to stay away from them. Some smells make us shudder, some make us turn away, some just smell horrible. Any given perfume may delight one person and offend another. There is no accounting for taste—or smell. We also may find something disgusting simply because we have had too much of it.

I don't like most commercial perfume, although I enjoy pure essential oils, especially when they are unmixed. Many years ago I used to love incense, but for the last 20 years or so I've disliked almost all of it. There are only a few impossible-to-get varieties that I can still tolerate. What I sometimes do is take one stick of incense I like and leave it out, unlit. To me, that hint of a sacred smell says more than a houseful of smoke.

Sensitizing yourself to smell makes you more aware of environments you might not want to be in. If you can, give yourself a choice to follow those cues rather than make your body stay in a place that does not smell good to you.

Explore What Disgusts You

Go find something disgusting to your sense of smell. It could be anything: window cleaner, a corner of the garage, mildew, compost or fertilizer, or a perfume you do not like. Take a whiff and notice how your body reacts. You may have creepy sensations, and you will probably feel the urge to move away and turn your head away from the source of the smell. Honor this knowing.

Now consider: If you were to honor your sense of disgust, what changes would you make in your life? Is there some action you have been waiting to take that would make your world smell better? I gave up smoking not because my two cigarettes a day were so bad but because it was impossible to get the smell off. Even a shower, shampoo, and brushing my teeth twice a day would not get rid of the stench of tobacco. So I just let it go.

While writing this chapter, I found myself going through my closet and tossing more than half of my old clothes. I live near the ocean, and the things I never wear get musty. So I donated them to Goodwill. Cleanse your life of smells you find disgusting and notice how you feel.

A related exercise is to find something that you think smells disgusting and talk to someone who likes it. My friend Ilene loves the smell of horse stables and cigarette stubs. To her they both mean that someone has been having a good time: Horse manure indicates riding, and cigarette stubs suggest that people may have been sitting around talking up a storm. If you ask around, you may discover some amazing smells you never dreamed of enjoying.

You also could explore smells that you associate with cleansing. The scent of bleach might be acrid, but it is a relief to smell when something mildewed is nearby. Some American Indian tribes use the smoke of burning cedar, sage, or pine needles to purify a place. Companies that make cleaning solutions seem to agree that pine is a cleansing smell.

I remember the first time someone offered me sips of single-malt scotch. One tasted like iodine—ugh—and one tasted like burnt weeds. But I've come to love scotch, and although I don't drink it very often (maybe twice a year) just thinking about those initially disgusting tastes is somehow very enlightening.

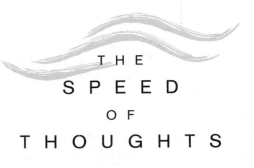

THE
S P E E D
O F
T H O U G H T S

*D*uring your breathwork you'll notice the *speed* of thoughts coming and going, each with an emotional charge. This is one of the main things students of breath complain about: A thought will come, and before it has a chance to unfold, a different thought comes along. There is a whole battery of thoughts with every breath and they move as fast as a television commercial! To get what I mean, watch television and note how quickly the scenes shift. The individual shots are designed to last a split second less than your attention span. Watch different kinds of movies. Action/adventure flicks are driven by quick cuts, while the shots in dramas and most comedies are held longer, to develop a more complicated narrative. And any film from the 1940s or 1950s, you'll notice, moves at a much slower pace.

Your mental reaction time is fast. So when an emotion arises, you may find yourself quickly starting to block it. That might be appropriate in a business meeting, but not in a meeting with yourself. The process seems messy, but if you breathe with the emotion, the brain will sort things out.

Again, your mental reaction time is fast. Lean into the speed of your thoughts and feelings. Tell your brain to go for it. Let it race as fast as it wants to. Over the course of a few conscious breaths or a few minutes of breathing, you will notice that you have created enough space to feel the feelings. And that is what healing is all about.

Slow Down

Western society worships speed, and the pace of modern everyday life gets faster all the time. There is definitely something wonderful about that. And yet much enjoyment can be had in very slow, languorous motion.

First, take a few moments to settle down, to slow down. Then, sit down and engage yourself. Rest your palms in your lap and move one finger; then move it more slowly; then move it so slowly that you can't tell just by looking at it whether it is moving or not.

Move your head in a way that would be invisible to someone

watching but perceptible to you. Keep this slow motion going for a minute, then let it fade away.

Move your head forward and back as in the Explore Up and Down exercise on page 37. Then, slowly, over a period of several minutes, let the motion coast to stillness. As the motion becomes less physically pronounced, the subjective sensation of motion may increase because you have become so alert to subtle kinesthesia. When you finally become still, the sense of motion increases even more, so you have a sense of stillness-in-motion. In this way, even just sitting still becomes very interesting.

If you like, practice your favorite sport or hobby in slow motion. Then slower motion. Then slo-o-o-o-ow motion.

WHERE
DOES YOUR
MIND GO
WHEN IT
WANDERS?

*W*hen you are doing a task and your mind wanders, where

does it go?

Sexual fantasies	Children
Job worries	Incomplete projects
Lovers and relationships	Creative ideas

These mental journeys may occur whenever you have a

moment to yourself, even if it is just for the space of a

breath. This happens because you have relaxed and are set-

tling into your body. You are becoming aware of your needs.

When your mind wanders, it is showing you something.

Whatever scene you are thinking about is designed to re-

mind you to enjoy yourself. Even if you are thinking of

things you feel tense about, the wandering is there to help you find a way through the obstacles so you can enjoy yourself again.

Your nervous system is always seeking to bring itself up to date, into the now. It wants to reflect on experiences you have had, let nonessential things fade into the background, get a good plan together for the future, and update its map of the world. When your mind wanders, this is what it's doing. It's processing information.

When you pay attention to the breath, no matter how earnest you are, your mind will wander. But don't be concerned because this wandering is in the service of life. It is part of the process. If you think, *My mind is wandering, I have to concentrate harder*, you will miss the spontaneous intelligence arising from within you.

One day, a very loving woman who is a grandmother came over for a session. She sat down and I invited her to pay attention to her breath. After a couple of minutes, she apologized because her mind was wandering. She said that she was thinking of one of her grandchildren who was going through a tough time. I told her that what she was doing was bringing that little girl into the space of her meditation and breathing a blessing on her. Her mind was not wandering; rather, it was very purposeful.

The basic principle is this: *Life moves.* Life goes after the fulfillment of needs. When you enter the world of your breathing, you will witness this movement, which is usually subliminal. Accept each thought, each impulse as a blessing, and bless it in return. Even though you crave peace and want rest and silence right now, accept the yearnings that arise in your heart and everywhere in your being.

Follow Your
Wandering Mind

Sometimes we find ourselves thinking of somewhere we would rather be—in a different situation or a far-off place. We may believe that if we were elsewhere, we could be breathing easily. The purpose of this exercise is to remind you to get up and go to that place now, to remind you that you could, or to suggest that you can work to improve your situation right here and now.

Where does your mind wander if you give it the chance? What do you start thinking about? Right now, take a minute to enjoy your breathing. As you do, note what thoughts come and go through the back of your mind. Give yourself total permission to wander the world of your experience. What is it reminding you of?

Maybe you are able to pay attention to your breathing for the first 2 minutes and then your mind wanders: You are standing on a beach in Tahiti, drinking some tropical drink with a colorful little paper umbrella in it. Maybe you saw a similar scene in an ad in the newspaper or a magazine, or maybe you are remembering your honeymoon. Perhaps this is just a longing you have; pay attention to it. Explore your desire, whether it is to sit in a café in Paris drinking good coffee, to stand on top of a Himalayan mountain breathing the thin, cold air, or to lie down in a field by a stream you know and listen to the wind in the trees.

When you feel that the thought is finished, let your attention shift back to the physical sensations of breath.

The job of paying attention is to say, *I am here. Tell me the truth. What is going on?* and then listening. The goal of paying attention is to tolerate the truth.

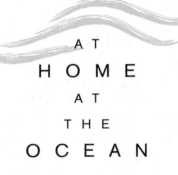

AT
HOME
AT
THE
OCEAN

I grew up at the beach in southern California, smelling the brine and the sweet weeds on the cliffs, the wild mustard and anise. To me, the smell of air that has blown my way over thousands of miles of ocean is the smell of home.

Many of my friends think that the Coast is okay but prefer to live inland, in New Mexico and eastward. I am littoral. I'd pine away for the ocean if I lived anywhere else.

In fact, my friend Michael and I shaped the basic ideas of this book during long swims off Malibu. We generally would venture about a mile north or south from a given point and then walk back. Sometimes we would pause out there in the water and get into a whole discussion; sometimes we would pull up to a convenient rock, one that the seals were not occupying at the moment, and talk all afternoon. Often it was as we were walking back along the beach and through rocky coves, thoroughly at home with ourselves and breathing deeply the ocean air, that our concepts about breath came to be spoken in words above the roar of the surf.

Many modern men and women go about the business of their lives detached from their environments. They are homeless in their own homes, even in their own bodies. Americans move a lot. They work a lot. When they finally do come home, it's likely that they'll sit down in front of the television.

For all of our material possessions, too many of us don't know how to inhabit our living spaces, our little corners of the world, and make them our own.

Make Yourself
at Home

Step outside for a moment, or make a daytrip to where the air is fresh, and take a deep breath. Then bring something that smells good back inside your house or apartment. The smell does not have to be strong. You might have a single coffee bean, one leaf, an orange rind, or a dab of peppermint oil on a piece of paper. This helps particularly if you are living in a place that does not feel like home to you.

If you already feel at home in your living space but would like it to feel even homier, put something on to cook.

While writing this chapter I found myself hankering for good smells. So I went to the store and bought cookie mix and cinnamon-roll mix, and every afternoon for a few days I baked. The smells made me happy. I live in an apartment building, and when people would walk by my door, I would sometimes hear them say *"Mmmmmm."* I would take breaks from writing and walk around with a tray of either chocolate-chip cookies or hot cinnamon rolls, offering them to my neighbors, the postman, the gardeners, and anyone else who happened by. It took only a few minutes to prepare the mixes, a short time in the oven, and not long at all to give them away, but I got to live with incredible smells for hours, and this really brightened my days.

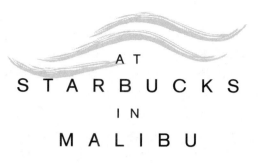

AT
STARBUCKS
IN
MALIBU

On my way to swim in Malibu, I often stop and have a cup
of coffee at Starbucks, which attracts a colorful crowd. There
are glamorous women, trophy wives in jodhpurs, scruffy canyon
denizens, scriptwriters with laptops, surfers, and occasionally a
homeless person or a movie star.

There is a marked contrast between those who come in,
sit down, and slowly sip their drinks, and the majority,
who come and go hastily, carrying their drinks out to their
cars—an assortment of shiny new SUVs, too many Land
Rovers that have never been off the pavement, BMWs, and
one or two old trucks. The coffee-to-go crowd is breath-
less. It is as if they take it as a matter of status that they have

no time to enjoy their drinks. And most do not drink just plain coffee; they order cappuccinos that are as luxurious as chocolate milk shakes, with something like 15 different tastes dancing on your tongue with any given sip.

I don't know anyone who can properly enjoy a cup of coffee or even really taste it while driving. Especially on a strip of road like in Malibu, where cars drive at freeway speed only a foot or two from parked cars, pedestrians, and surfers carrying boards.

The lesson in this story: Give yourself more time to taste.

Wake Up
to the Smell of Your Coffee

When you imbibe your daily pleasure, whether peppermint tea, apple juice, water, sports drink, coffee, espresso, or soda, pay total attention and give yourself time to inhale the smell while you slowly sip. Cultivate the feeling that you are inhaling the scent into your body and directly absorbing energy and stimulation. The smell, the moisture, the taste—when they enter you, they activate you. The invisible, ethereal essence of the substance goes into your system and feeds you. Cherish the stimulation.

Hold the cup in both hands. Lift it up and hold it under your nose for a moment and inhale. Then take a sip, and let your awareness be completely in your tongue and around the inside of your mouth. Breathe out slightly, directing the air over your tongue, and see if this amplifies the taste. Then take a breath.

Coffee, tea, or even water can be nourishing, soothing, and exciting, all at the same time. I often drink tap water that has been run through a filter, and it is most delicious.

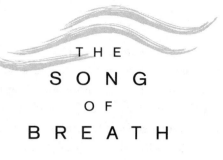

THE
SONG
OF
BREATH

*W*hen we breathe, we make sounds: There is a general whoosh of air, along with spontaneous and incidental *oooh*s and *ahhh*s. Although we generally ignore these sounds, if we listen closely we can learn a lot from them.

The song of our breath will change its tune according to our actions and emotions. When we are being quiet, the breath comes very softly (pianissimo). When we walk fast or run, it hurries along in brisk and lively fashion (allegro). When we are feeling strong emotions, the breath also becomes loud and strong (forte). By monitoring the tempo of our breath, we can somewhat gauge our temper.

The sounds of breath we pay the most attention to are

the shaped sounds—human speech. (Note that all speech origi-
nates in the exhalation. It is possible to speak on the inhalation,
but it is difficult and rather ridiculous sounding.) However, as a
conscious breather you should set yourself the task of knowing
and loving all the dimensions of breathing sounds, from the spontaneous exclamations—"Argh!" "O-o-oh!" "Mmmmmm . . ." —to
chanting, whispers, and the most eloquent speech. For instance,
when we breathe in forcefully, the sound might be called
snorting. But think of the breath of an athlete running, or of a
couple making love. The huffing, the puffing, the grunting provides a beautiful soundtrack for life's simple pleasures.

Listening to breath should be like listening to music. Do not
just use your ears; listen with your whole body. The vibrations
of the music—no matter what kind or how loud it is—touch
our skin and vibrate our internal organs. Some music makes the
heart sing, some makes us want to wiggle or shake, some moves
us to tears, some lifts us up. Part of the pleasure of music is savoring these sensations throughout the body as we listen. We
can appreciate the song of breath in the same way.

Listen to the Sounds of Breath

While sitting, take a few deep breaths and notice the sounds the
air makes as it flows through the different parts of your body—
your nose, sinuses, and throat. Open your mouth slightly and enjoy
the sounds of the air as it touches your lips and tongue. Alternately
speed up and slow down your breathing, and simply explore in a
childlike way the different sounds that are produced and feelings
that are evoked. You may find some of them particularly charming.

Even 1 minute of this can leave you feeling refreshed and energized, and it's a good way to start any meditation. Over time you will learn to enjoy more and more subtle differentiations. Just as at a party you can selectively listen to different conversations, within your body you can learn to selectively hear many different nuances of breathing sounds.

Follow your sense of pleasure, shifting the tempo as you like, from slow to fast and everywhere in between. Sometimes you will find yourself falling into very subtle breathing and other times you will find yourself craving fast breath, with all of the intense sensations that go with it. You will never know what cravings you will have for a particular tempo of breath until you are absorbed in the exploration.

After satisfying your craving for speed or slowness, allow yourself to rest in these breath sounds. Then, let your attention drift away and just rest in yourself for a moment before opening your eyes.

Variations:

➤ If you want to make your exercise program more entertaining, do a few minutes of listening to the sounds of breath as a meditation, then jump up and go walking or running, go to the gym, or play your favorite sport. Carry the appreciation of breath sound with you as you move.

➤ Seek out a place that is very quiet: the desert, an empty church, or anywhere at 4:00 A.M., and listen to the quiet sounds that even the subtlest breath produces. As you gradually inhabit your body more and more in the silence, you may learn to hear the organic sounds of the air flowing through the sinus caverns in your head, and you may feel and hear the air moving behind your eyes and your ears. You can hear the rhythm of air, the river of air. Listen to the river of air moving in a circular way. It resonates throughout your whole upper torso.

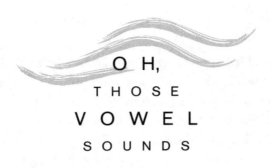

O H,
T H O S E
V O W E L
S O U N D S

*T*here is a wonderful scene in *The Wizard of* Oz where the Wicked Witch's army is marching and chanting, "Oh EE oh . . . Yo-oh. Oh EE oh . . . Yo-oh." The voices are sincere, deep, and yet kid-friendly. One year my nieces—four of them under the age of 6—watched the video over and over and would tromp around, intoning the vowels with immense delight.

If you have ever heard work songs, children singing nonsense syllables to themselves, or Gregorian or Tibetan chanting, then you may appreciate the continuum of wonderful sounds we humans can make. And some of the most deeply pleasing utterances are the sounds of the vowels: a, e, i, o, and u. Even if you are not a singer, you can chant the vowel sounds, at least to yourself. When you whisper, the vowel sounds will resonate in you, soothe you, energize you, and feed you.

When you do the simple vowel sound breathing exercises that follow, you will find that your sense of hearing is heightened. In this way, listening to your inner music makes you more appreciative of outer music.

Mouth the
Vowel Sounds

Do this exercise both sitting up and lying down. It is quite different in each position.

Begin by whispering the vowel sounds. Just get the sense of what it is like to sit or lie down by yourself and whisper. Do this for 10 exhalations.

Now allow your vocal cords to come into play so that you are actually speaking the vowel sounds. Feel the particular vibration of each vowel and try to identify where in your body it resonates. Explore all of the vowel sounds both in your native tongue and in any other language you know.

Then select your favorite two vowels and breathe out with them again and again. Delight in them, as a child would.

Now sustain the sound, like the background chorus of a song. Think of R&B groups with their backup singers doing their *oo-wah*s. It really adds something to the texture of the music. When you learn to listen to the vowels, you add something to the soundtrack of your life.

By mouthing the vowel sounds with different stresses, tones,

volume, and rhythm, you can make them soothing, exhilarating, healing, passionate, or haunting. The vowel sounds possess all of these qualities, and as you get familiar with what your
personal range is, you can draw out every nuance. One of my
favorite practices is resting in the vowel sounds, which can
bring on a profoundly restful and energizing meditation.
Resting in this case means that you chant for a few minutes,
then ease off and just listen to the echoes for a while, allowing
the resonance of the sounds to continue. This is a good technique to do for 5 minutes every morning. It will relax your
voice for the day, clear your head, and wake you up.

Act Out
Primal Speech

What you are about to do here is reenact the evolution of
speech—in a hurry.

Start by pretending to be a caveman or cavewoman having a
conversation with a friend using only grunts and groans. See
how much information you can convey about how your day
went. Include sounds such as keening, moaning, or cooing, that
are meant to express how you are feeling inside. (For reference,
you might try listening to recordings of wolves howling or orcas
breathing before doing this exercise.)

Look at things in your environment and make up word-
sound names for them, such as *woof* for dog, *meow* for cat, *moo*
for cow, *bzzz* for bee, and so on. Master the feeling that you can
name things with sounds.

Gradually, let your sounds become more like speech. Finally,
shift to speaking as the most mannered Englishman you have

ever heard and read a section of the King James Version of the Bible or some exquisite poetry.

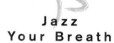

Jazz
Your Breath

Here you are going to play your breath like an instrument. And I do mean play!

Open your mouth and let the air flow out, then gently suck it back in. Purse your lips as if you were whistling or blowing smoke rings. Breathe in and out primarily though your mouth in a rhythmic, pulsing pattern. Do not hyperventilate—if you get dizzy, stop. Then try again more gently. If you still feel uncomfortable, discontinue.

Now pretend that you are a jazz musician blowing notes. Shape your mouth and utter the sounds "oooh," "hoo," "shaaa," "shhhhh," and "chaaa". Use these word-sounds as a basic vocabulary and make up your own as you go along. You will find that by changing the shape of your lips, you can change the sound, and you start to feel like you are playing some sort of weird, pulsing, breath instrument. On each exhalation, pull your belly in rapidly, forcing the air out. This gives you extra stimulation in the torso and in the mouth.

Now take a rest. (Jazz musicians are always taking 5.) Pause and notice the sensations. You may feel tingling, light-headedness, or energy flowing in your body.

Now resume. This time vary the rhythm and tempo of your exhalations, as though you were riffing on the basic melody.

ACTIVATING
YOUR
ENERGY
CENTERS

*T*he human body is a system of energy centers where

nerve and blood pathways meet and intertwine. In

anatomy, such a center is called a plexus, a word that

means a combination of interlaced parts, or a network.

You can feel in your body where these centers are because

you are more sensitive there, you have feeling there. The

cardiac or heart plexus is not just where your blood is

pumped and oxygenated—you can feel emotions there;

the solar plexus is not just your pancreas, it's where you

feel butterflies in your stomach; and the pelvic plexus is

richly supplied with the nerves and blood vessels we take

such delight in when we engage in sex or even think about

it. There are dozens of major and minor plexi throughout the body, and they all can contribute to your enjoyment of breathing.

These energy centers, called chakras in Sanskrit, have long been known to the mystic traditions of India, Tibet, China, and Japan and are addressed in meditation, martial arts, and certain healing practices. The energy that extends out from the body— magnetic tinglings that you can feel in the space around you— is called your aura. If you don't believe in this concept, you don't need to explore it in depth. Simply consider it your sense of proximity.

The approach to take is to luxuriate in each center. Don't work hard at it. Always follow your bodily hunches with regard to exploring your energy centers, and don't force anything. The centers are sofas—places where attention can rest. They are also pivotal places where work is done, where what is inside you meets the world, where energy comes in and nurtures you or poisons you, and where energy exits the body.

The heart, for example, is a center of nerves and blood vessels. So are the sexual organs. But both also field very strong relational feelings.

There are two broad categories of energy-center sensations.

1. Sensations in the head, throat, chest, belly, genitals, hands, feet, and other areas of the body that are nerve plexi or chakras

2. Those that cause magnetic, tingling, electrical, or energetic sensations; this is the "subtle body," the pranamayakosha, the chi, the aura

The energy centers feel as if they breathe—as if something, some subtle essence in air, some force, can flow in and out of each center. This is a very invigorating, purifying, and enlightening sensation.

And yet there are many reasons why you may not be open to such subtle sensations. You may not feel safe enough to allow yourself to be so sensitive, or your body may be preparing you for such an awakening in exactly 2 years but for now you can't help but focus on the concrete.

Regardless of why, if you do not have such a sensation, do not waste even 1 second worrying about it. Just go through the motions of one of the following exercises. If you still don't connect with your energy centers, or if you don't like the sensations that you connect with, move on and try again—in a week, a month, or a year.

Lay Your Hands On—Yourself

Breathe for a few minutes with your bodily sensations and emotions. Then place the palms of your hands together over your chest. If you pray, say your favorite prayer for healing and guidance. Hold your hands there for a few breaths, then let one hand move up and rest on your forehead and the other move down and rest on your pelvic bone, just below your belly button. In doing this, you will tend over time to become aware of the space *between* your hands, as if each palm has a different polarity and a current flows between them. Pay attention to the current flowing between your pelvis and your head. Chances are, you will find it pleasurable.

After a minute or two, let one hand move to your heart and the other to your belly. Breathe with your palms in that position, feeling with close attention the emotions, currents, and sensations that are vibrating through you. As you get used to this, begin to notice and explore different parts of your torso: under the ribs; the solar plexus area, around the navel, the pubic bone. Feel the inner space of the pelvic bowl, inside the hipbones. These are areas that are massaged by breath, and interestingly, they are also areas of emotional connection to others. When we hug people, we reach out and take them into the warm and protective circle of our arms. When we make love, we welcome our beloved into very close bodily contact.

You will have to be alert to your internal flows so that your energies can refresh themselves through fluctuation. Be open to your needs. If you have a rule that sleep is bad during the breath exploration, you may prevent yourself from resting deeply or even sleeping. This may leave you tired and irritable. If you have a rule against entertaining erotic feelings, you may block the flow of energy through your pelvis, and from there to the whole body. Sexual energy is a zesty form of the life force, and in general it is very healing. Your challenge will be to not let your learned resistance interfere with your ability to pay attention. Accept your fear and bless it.

As your senses develop and you get used to the subtle currents flowing in you, consider where in your body you might not have enough energy. What parts of your heart, your belly, your throat, your head, or your pelvis have become depleted? Just by paying attention during the laying on of hands, balance and flow will be restored. What parts of your body are congested with too much energy? As you practice this technique, your sense of pleasure will guide you. The laying on of hands is self-regulating and should feel like a catnap that leaves you refreshed. In this way you develop instincts for healing yourself and balancing your energy centers. It is similar to the mending process that happens when we sleep, except that we are conscious and participating.

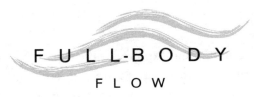

FULL-BODY
FLOW

Anyone can have an excessive concentration of energy in their energy centers. When you focus your attention on those areas, you may feel heat, intensity, tension, pain, or fatigue. If you are a loving person and you lose a partner, your heart may become congested with excess energy— you ache to let your love flow. If you are physically passionate, your pelvis may become congested and you will ache to let your sexual energy flow. Other energy centers will call out in different ways if neglected. Instead of being congested, they are hungry for attention. As a result, they feel empty, numb, cold. You can, with your hands and through breath awareness, channel excess energy to those needy centers so that full-body balance is restored.

Marianne, a schoolteacher friend of mine, describes her experience with breath this way:

> In the afternoon or early evening, I take time for myself. I lie down, place my hands on my abdomen, and pay attention to my breathing. I notice where in my body the breath is flowing and where it isn't. I place my hands on where it is not flowing and just stay there, attentive, for a few minutes, until the feeling of breath flowing is restored. Usually, there is something I have to face—some issue, a feeling, a person, a thought I lost track of during the bustle of the day. I have to be willing to face something and feel something; then I have my body back. I can inhabit myself again. The whole thing takes between a half-hour and an hour. Afterward, I am refreshed, not a worn-out servant of humanity limping through the evening. I'm full of life and ready for trouble.

The decision to take time out of your busy day like this is all about quality. When you allow yourself maintenance time, you will be more available to life.

Another friend, Rob, somehow finds the time to meditate every day after work even though he has two teenage sons with whom he is very involved. This is what he told me:

> At some point in the evening I find a place to lie down, usually in the living room. I put my hands on my belly or on my heart and I take the breath into me. That one breath is different somehow from all the unconscious breaths before it—it is the breath of God, and I cherish it. I take it in as if it is the healing substance of the universe, and man, do I need it. Then what happens is my

attention transfers into my body. All day long, my attention is on what everyone else needs—my customers, my boss, the owners of the company, my wife, the kids, the car, the teachers at school, my friends. This is the one time in my day where I can let my attention truly rest in my body, and the sensation is wild—I feel incredible release, an almost sexual gushing, and I would start laughing except I am too tired to move.

I feel a tingling afterward. It is kind of a furry feeling, a fur made out of warm energy.

Do a Daily Emotion Scan

Sit or lie down; get comfortable. If possible and appropriate, turn off the phone. Let a minute go by.

Become aware of your body as it exists in the midst of your life. Notice the time and place: *I am home, it is 6 o'clock on Tuesday evening; my wife is in the other room, my kids are off at college.* Or, *It is 9 o'clock Saturday morning; I have half an hour to myself before going to meet my friends.*

Be aware of your body as relatively still, with mainly the breath moving. Allow any background tension to come to the foreground. Anything you are nervous about or have mixed feelings about, let it come up. Such thoughts will come, whether you welcome them or not, so why not be hospitable? Greet each worry and give it a bath or a shower or a massage in breath. You do this by allowing the thought to bother you and then sinking deeper and deeper into breath awareness, so that you marshal the resources of calmness and acceptance to deal with the thoughts and emotions to be healed.

Keep scanning your body—belly, chest, throat, forehead—for sensations that go with any emotions you may be experiencing. Being available to these emotions is the key to self-healing.

Sometimes the sensations need a lot of attention before they can be released. For example, you may not be able to shake your feelings of anger for someone at work. You may feel in your arms and chest a strong desire to hit. In this case you'll need to explore the way in which anger is striking out.

When our feelings are hurt, we are hurt and may experience this as an ache. Grief may feel like a sinking down; loneliness like a sense of being disconnected from the wholeness of life. Everyone's sensations are different. Notice what you feel as you lie or sit there, breathing and taking it all as it comes.

This kind of emotion scan is about catching yourself as you are. Ideally, you are being the best friend, the best lover, that a person could want—to yourself. You are there, tender and loving, for yourself as an emotional human being. As a bonus, when you make the time to do a daily emotion scan, you wind up doing volunteer work for the world. It is as if you have a garden and you wind up feeding the neighborhood, keeping everyone in tomatoes and lettuce, because you do the work of weeding, plowing, planting, watering, and harvesting. Like gardening, it's a lot of work and a lot of joy.

Develop a series of emotion scans ranging from a few seconds to a few hours. Although you might start out sitting or lying down, you could also learn how to scan while walking or doing some other physical exercise. Your time could be on weekends, when you go to a special place. At the very least, get into the habit of a daily 5-minute scan. When you come home, lie down for 5 minutes and simply notice the coming and going of thoughts. Give attention to whatever emotions call to you. Then notice if you don't feel better all evening.

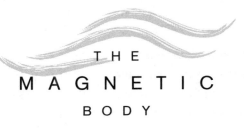

THE
M A G N E T I C
B O D Y

*A*s you learn to pay attention to the breath in your
body, your senses will unfold and you will find that
you are able to refresh yourself at will. But there is a
whole other realm of sensations to be explored in connection with breath and the energy centers. I am never sure
what to call this realm because the names given to it—the
aura, the subtle body, the pranamayakosha—are so
grandiose that they take away from its immediacy and sensuality. The sensations themselves are usually tiny and
variable.

- Slight tingling sensations
- A feeling of magnetism in and around the body
- Currents of some kind of energy flowing in the body
- A sense that the air is full of some kind of charged particles

➤ The sensation that space is almost solid and solids are space

➤ Feeling the space around the body extend out
to a distance of 3 to 5 feet

These sensations are often felt on the surface of the skin, or even in the space surrounding the skin. I tend to call this realm of subtle-body perceptions *the magnetic body*.

If you are already experiencing such subtle energies, it will be a relief to do the following explorations. It will be a treat, like taking a shower after working out. But not everyone feels these energies all the time. When I conduct these exercises in breath workshops, sometimes only about half of my students feel sure that they've touched their magnetic bodies.

That being said, give these exercises a chance. Exploring your magnetic body is very simple. All you need to do is move your hands in and out from your body—the basic in-and-out motion of breathing—as if there is some subtle substance or energy that you are imbibing directly into your body. This energy has qualities of luminosity, vibrancy, nutrition, healing, music, color, and sometimes, magic. It is the feeling that people talk about when they say that something is "thrilling" or "inspired" or "radiant."

Many senses come into play when you are sensing this kind of energy—temperature, very light touch, joint sensing, motion sensing, and sometimes vision and hearing. Some people claim that they can see this energy; others say that they can hear it vibrating.

In any case, it is most important to not impose anything on yourself. If you do not feel anything today, you might tomorrow, or in a year. Trust your body. There is more than enough to keep track of in this world without being overly concerned with subtle energies.

Breathe
Magnetism

You can do this exercise anytime you feel tuned in and sensitive. You can be standing or sitting, outside or inside.

With your hands extended slightly away from your body and your palms facing each other, rest in your breathing. Allow the movement of the breath to support your arms as they levitate.

Become curious about what is there between your palms. Move your palms in toward your heart as you breathe in, and move them away as you breathe out. Continue in this way for about 5 minutes and notice what happens. You may begin to feel as if there is a subtle energy that flows directly into your heart—the energy of breath. In terms of magnetism, this is true—there is a streaming quality through the heart when it is open. You are letting your heart breathe magnetism.

My students describe the kind of energy they are sensing as:

Charging	Protective	Peaceful
Inspiring	Nurturing	Strong
Electrifying	Purifying	Exciting
Soothing		

You can see several opposites here, in particular the dimensions of soothing-exciting and nurturing-purifying. My impression is that these polarities tend to change every 15 to 45 seconds. As soon as you get used to the qualities of one mode, it changes to another. This is how life refreshes itself—through a continual oscillation between the complementary tones of resting and being excited, feeding and purifying, homing and exploring. If you enjoy this exercise, come back to it every day and explore it in depth for yourself.

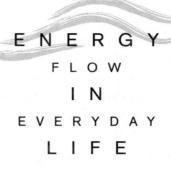

ENERGY
FLOW
IN
EVERYDAY
LIFE

*Y*ou may not have energy sensitivity. If not, that's fine. But many people have intuition or clairvoyance without realizing it, and it's a problem for them until they learn to live with it. It's a bit like having a pet; if you don't feed it and care for it, there will be problems. Perceptual gifts need to be acknowledged and heeded, then massaged, groomed, and rested. They require almost as much maintenance as a dog. Maybe more.

When you take the time to attend to the energy flows in and around your body, you are cleaning the sensory-pathways and energy circuits that your body uses to nourish what is called intuition.

The energy centers, or chakras, correspond with your nerve plexi; it is here that the dimensions of breath—metabolism, information, and emotion—meet and greet one another. The centers evolve according to how you give and receive energy from the world. In general, they can be developed through regular use. For example, if you want to evolve your heart chakra, you should be fully involved in the play of expressing your love in the outer world, and then be able to withdraw into yourself and re-create this effect. Energy always involves the interplay of inner and outer.

In fact, opening the chakras and closing them should be taught together. The New Age practitioners who have adopted parts of the ancient teachings tend to emphasize opening the chakras and purifying them. This is out of balance. You always want to be able to open *and* to close. Also, purification generally takes care of itself, so it is better to put your attention on nourishing your energy centers. Nurture your heart, your solar plexus area, and your pelvis. Nurturing awareness is instinctively satisfying.

You don't need to try to create energy centers that aren't there, either. If you don't feel anything, it may just mean that there is nothing wrong. You don't feel much in your knee unless you have injured it or overused it. The same goes for chakras.

If you impose the generic chakra system upon yourself, it may obliterate your own sensations. This could have a strong effect, making it harder for you to know what you feel and more difficult for you to access your intuition. You also risk never feeling at home in your own body.

I love knowing about the chakras, and I regard their mapping as something exquisite—the yoga traditions have assigned sounds, colors, and elements for each. But in actual practice, knowing that you have chakras is like knowing you have pupils in your eyes. They take care of themselves, adapting to conditions as needed.

Explore the
Palms of Your Hands

You can do this while standing or sitting. Eventually, you should try it both ways so you can discover your preference.

If you are sitting, rest your palms in your lap for a minute and simply be aware of them. Rest in your breathing. Be aware of the enchanting quality of breath, its magic.

If you are standing, let your hands dangle at your sides, and then become aware of them.

Turn your palms to face each other. Position them about 1½ feet apart or whatever you find comfortable. Experiment with increasing and decreasing that distance and notice the sensations that arise as you do so. Notice the empty space between your palms.

As you bring your hands closer together, what do you feel? As you move your hands away from each other, what sensations arise? You might immediately start having tiny tingling sensations, you might experience nothing for 5 minutes and then start to feel warm, or something else entirely might come up.

Draw your hands toward your belly. If you let your elbows be at your sides with your forearms pointing forward, your hands will be at about belly level. Find a comfortable pose there. Turn your hands to face your belly button and then focus on your breathing.

After a minute, let your hands move in and out slightly with your breath—about a half-inch of motion. It is unusual to move so slowly, so if this feels awkward, be gentle with yourself and do not push. Continue this way for 5 minutes or, if you get uncomfortable, stop and come back another time.

Breathe energy into your heart. Raise your hands to the level of your heart and move your arms out slightly, as if your hands and arms were helping to draw the air in and push it out. Move your hands in and out, gently following the breath, for about 5 minutes. Get into the ebb and flow of it. Very often for a beginner, within that period of time you may begin to feel something. If you do feel the energy flowing, meaning you have interesting sensations in your hands and heart, then continue as long as you like. Play with the energy. This is similar to the Breathe Magnetism exercise on page 118. In this exploration, simply focus on the sense of flow and pleasure. Give yourself a chance to discover a style and pace of hand motions that are so pleasurable that they begin to come spontaneously.

If you do not feel anything within 5 minutes, stop and come back to this exploration another day. Perhaps wait until some sunny afternoon in a park or at a lake or in a forest.

If you start to feel something and want to explore more of the vocabulary of movement, there are many tai chi videotapes and classes available.

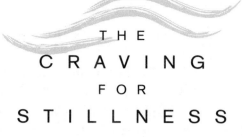

THE
C R A V I N G
F O R
S T I L L N E S S

*B*usy people often have a deep craving for stillness.

They want their minds and their emotions to be still, at

least for a few moments of peace. Because the concept of

breath control originated within the ancient discipline of

yoga, which traditionally has been practiced by reclusive

monks, those seeking stress relief may think that the way

to a quiet mind is to block out their thoughts, squelch

their desires, and cultivate a sense of detachment from the

real world. It doesn't help that many breath-control ex-

perts are so absorbed in teaching the ancient techniques

that they don't allow for the fact that their students

do live in the real, noisy world and don't have the

spiritual luxury of meditating alone in a cave before, during, or after their classes.

True, it is hard to tolerate the craving for silence. But if you breathe *with* the craving rather than fight it, the breath will carry you into a living sense of stillness-in-motion. You just have to train yourself to tolerate the pain of the craving, which often feels bittersweet, like when your leg muscles are sore from walking too much.

If you can acknowledge your craving for stillness, and trust your breath to carry you through, you will have solace wherever you go.

Dance,
Then Lie Still

To do this exploration, first engage in movement of any kind that really pleases you—running, swimming, dancing, walking, climbing, anything that gets your breath rate and pulse up. Go for 5 minutes or so.

Then find a place to lie down and sense yourself.

For 1 minute, just let your mind wander. Then, begin to notice the breath without interfering with it in any way. You may notice that the breath is finding its own rhythm. It was faster, because you were moving, and now it is slowing down.

That's all. Simply witness the self-regulation of the breath rhythm.

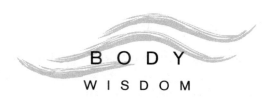

B O D Y
W I S D O M

*T*he way most of us live is not natural. Call it life in

the age of anxiety or whatever you want—we exist in a

state of minor panic about imagined or potential threats.

This kind of tension does not compute to the instinctive

self. The body would rather free its breathing from past

emotions and just breathe appropriately for the here and

now. If you are being targeted by a charging water buffalo,

your body wants to respond within $\frac{1}{10}$ of a second and be

in full flight, breathing as deeply as is humanly possible to

send huge gusts of oxygen to your muscles. If there is no

clear and present danger, however, your body would prefer

to be in absolute relaxation, conserving energy for the

next real emergency. Conscious breath taking can help restore sanity to your life by realistically updating your map of the world and retraining your musculature to respond appropriately to danger—and the lack thereof.

As students of breath, we may consciously want to be more calm, but our body wisdom is not interested in calmness per se. It is interested in accuracy of response, which means minimal expenditure of energy to accomplish a given task or confront a particular emotion. The more readily you accept this function of the body—which really is a function of the breath—the more calm you will feel from breath awareness because you are not trying to force anything or put anything over on your instinctive nervous system.

I know people who have practiced breath awareness for years and have developed a layer of calmness on top of their emotional life. It is as if they have used breath control to lay down linoleum over their raw, messy emotions and gut feelings. This mind-body split suggests that the real world and the spiritual world are utterly, irrevocably separate. They are not.

The primary challenge of breathwork, however, is to tolerate relaxation, not fake it. When you relax, you let go of muscular tension, but you must really feel the effects of the tension first before it can be released. That is the goal. Only then have you created a situation where your body can shift wisely from combat mode into healing mode.

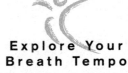

Explore Your Breath Tempo

In the modern world, you have to grow your own time. You have to establish your own tempo or you risk losing yourself in the hustle. Getting in touch with your breath can help you stay slightly ahead of the day's pace so that you're not bulldozed.

I am not suggesting that you should simply slow down, by the way. Rather, this exercise is all about developing a range of speeds so you can set your own pace for the day.

Notice what is. Count your breaths. How many breaths per minute are you taking? Use a clock or a stopwatch if you can. Do not slow your breathing down or speed it up, just enjoy it as it is and notice the tempo.

Breathe with your hands. With your hands at the level of your mouth, move them away as you exhale and toward your mouth as you inhale. Watch them and feel them. Do this for 1 full minute.

Breathe fast. Find a fast tempo you enjoy and breathe at that pace. Breathe as rapidly as you would while walking up a hill or running. Explore the sensations that arise.

Breathe slowly. Intentionally slow your breathing and note any changes in your body.

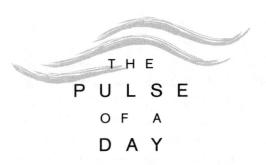

THE
PULSE
OF A
DAY

*T*here is a pulse to every day, a beat to which things move. It is dictated by our internal clocks, by how much rest we get, and by the time of day, the seasons, and the time in our lives we are in: childhood, adulthood, elderhood.

Sometimes we can consciously increase the tempo, although we may pay a heavy price. There are fiery debates about how much real work gets done when people hurry. Haste makes waste, the saying goes. Most of us acknowledge that there is a point beyond which we cannot push ourselves or our daily agendas. Indeed, one form of bullying that many of us are subjected to is the constant demands on our time. At work we may be given until noon to complete a job that would have taken an entire day 20 years ago.

Do you feel short on time or even starved for time? This is one of the curious paradoxes of life in the developed world. We have an abundance of things but a shortage of time. The industrialized world has given us access to more food of greater variety than ever before, more housing, better medicine, fewer infant deaths, less frequent outbreaks of disease, and greater knowledge of the universe. But we are poor in time. People report that they feel they have no time to see their friends, relax, smell the roses, meditate, or get to know themselves and their children. This comes from living at the pace of our machines rather than the pace of our breath.

Check the pulse of your here and now. Are you hurrying in any way as you read this? Do you want to get through the details to the real stuff? You may notice from time to time when reading that your eyes are urgently skipping over the surface of the text. I do this too, sometimes. The way out of this is simple—just allow the feeling of urgency to permeate you and breathe with it, and it will gradually change into excitement or relaxation.

When you do slow down, you may notice that you are flooded with anxious thoughts and feelings. That which you have been running from is now catching up with you. This is what you want—to catch up with yourself.

Lighten Up

When we are being responsible out in the world for the sake of our jobs and our families, we make ourselves "heavy" by doing what we need to do. That heaviness can persist when it's not necessary, and we can lose our ability to lighten up. Our posture can become slumped, as if we are dragging ourselves around. This exercise is intended to lighten you up by changing your perception of your body.

Imagine that your hands and feet are full of breath: light, buoyant, fluffy, transparent. There is no difference between the inside and the outside. Like balloons, your hands and feet are floating.

Now expand the scope of your play to lighten up completely.

- Picture your wrists filled with breath.
- Imagine that your elbows and the area under your armpits are filled with breath.
- Turn on "light" music and move gently to it.
- Let your feet sink down into the floor with just your hands floating upward.
- Imagine that the air inside your body and outside is the same.
- Feel the air flowing gently around your eyes, in your sinuses, and all around your face.
- What would it feel like if breath flowed into and out of your ears?
- Visualize your head as a helium balloon and your spine as a cord. Your head is floating free and buoyantly. If it might help, go get a helium balloon and bring it home to simulate the feeling.

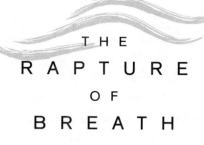

THE
R A P T U R E
O F
B R E A T H

Breathing in, I am conscious of rapture;
breathing out, I am conscious of rapture.

— B U D D H A

*B*reath is food, information, massage, delight, love, life,

and death. Breath is your healer and teacher. At any given

moment, your breath can correct any imbalance. Breath

connects the mind to the heart to the belly and integrates

the entire being with the soul. Breath unites us all and in-

vites us to experience that unity directly—if we are simply

aware of it.

Breath teaches us about life and death. The urge to

breathe in is the urge to live. Whenever you inhale, you

bring the stuff of creation into your body to meet your state of consciousness. Likewise, the urge to breathe out is the urge to die. There is stillness on both sides of breath.

What does breath have to do to food and water? It combines with and transforms them into spirit. Breath feeds the flame of life, continually transforming matter into spirit. What is metabolism anyway? Transformation from one thing into another.

Fill Yourself, and Empty

Breath is a continual rhythm of filling and emptying. As a metabolic function, it's about eating and excreting. You take something in, it gets transformed, and it is released.

Sit or lie down and simply pay attention to the feelings of being filled by breath and then being emptied. At first, be active. For about a minute, draw the air in and push it out with a bit of extra oomph. Then let go and be passive. Simply notice how the air flows in to fill you and flows out effortlessly without having to be manipulated in any way. If you are addicted to action, to making things happen, this is good for you to note.

This exercise seems mindlessly simple, and it is. But the dynamics of filling and emptying are fundamental to physical life, and both can be pleasurable. Also, any worries can be assuaged when you let your brain simplify the process of thoughts coming in and going out.

Get used to the idea of drawing nourishment out of the air.

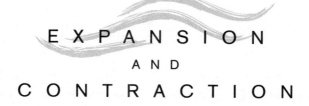

EXPANSION
AND
CONTRACTION

*P*hysically, during the act of breath taking, the skin of the belly and chest stretches slightly. From inside your lungs, you can feel your ribs pulling apart and drawing back together. But this expansion and contraction marks a more profound change in body structure as well.

When you expand, you take up a little more space in the world, you become a little more visible. Animals puff themselves up to appear larger. It is a daring thing, to expand.

When you contract, you condense yourself, so that you become smaller and less threatening to others.

Martha Graham, the world-famous dancer and choreographer, recognized this pulsation of expansion and contraction as one of the basic movements of life, and it informed her technique.

As you consciously engage with breath, get to know and love both expansion and contraction and work to continually extend your appreciation of each.

Do the Dance
of Expansion and Contraction

Stand with your arms at your sides. For a moment, notice the expansion and then contraction of your rib cage as you breathe in and out.

On the inhalation, your torso expands. Be with this expansion.

Now raise your arms in front of you and form a circle with your fingertips almost touching. Move your arms a little with the motion of your ribs. Let your ribs dictate to your arms, so when they expand, your arms expand. Inhale—spread wide; exhale—contract. This movement can be just a fraction of an inch, or you may feel like doing large movements. Continue the exercise until you settle into the subtle dance.

Stand with your arms at your sides again. Then spread your arms to each side, like a bird lifting its wings. Continue raising them up and over your head. After you experience this motion once, raise your arms above your head on the inhale and lower them on the exhale. Notice how this opens up your breathing.

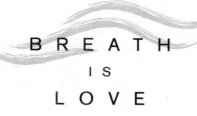

B R E A T H
I S
L O V E

*S*o much of loving is paying attention, cherishing, truly

listening, really taking the other person inside, and not

being defensive. You can learn much about all of this by

paying attention to the flow of breath.

"Attention is love," says the poet Marge Piercy. It seems

that when we truly pay attention, we tend to fall in love.

Love is a state of heightened appreciation, a condition in

which we do not take the other for granted. Appreciation

is to give value, and in love we give infinite value to the

beloved.

Breath is the movement of love, the interpenetration of

bodies—your body and the body of the Earth. To breathe

in is to receive love from the world and at the same time

literally extend life. To breathe out is to give love to the world, to share your essence. When you love someone, you want them to be close, to be part of your life. They are in your heart. You want to hold them in your arms tenderly. You may even want to share a breath with them. All this is happening between you and the planet, too, with each breath, for all breaths are shared breaths. To take a deep breath is to be in the same existential state as to receive love: You open up wide, you are moved, you receive the other, and you take the beloved into you and make them part of you.

The part of your body that receives the breath is the area around your heart. When your lungs fill with the incoming air, your heart center is being caressed, stimulated, nourished. You are bringing more circulation, more activity into the heart center. So all the issues of the heart get massaged as well. If you have experienced pain in a relationship, that hurt will be brought into awareness to be healed. Breath is the most gentle ointment of healing imaginable. Each breath encourages you to let go of fear, to let go into life, and to allow more circulation between yourself and the world.

Don't be surprised that as you open to breath you experience all the issues of a serious relationship: intimacy, sorrow, trust, generosity. These are issues of dependency and interdependency. We are more dependent upon breath than we ever will be on any human being. In fact, we are dependent upon the entire global ecosystem. This dependency can be terrifying, but there is no other way than to face the fear.

You are being asked with each inbreath to be generous to yourself, to feed on life more generously so that you can, in return, give more back. Breathing fully is one of the easiest ways to be generous to yourself. Life is generous to us, and receiving its abundance gratefully is the least we can do.

Experience Breath
as Love

Explore this while walking, lying down, sitting—any time you can give yourself over to your inner experience.

Receive love. Welcome the new air into your body as you inhale, just as you stand at the door to welcome friends or family into your home. Soak up the love and let it fill your whole being. Focus on your capacity to be filled with love.

Give love. As you exhale, say goodbye to the old air with gratitude and relief. Let your breath flow out and touch your family, your friends, and everything you care about. Focus on your ability to let go, to release, and to give. As you exhale, give yourself to the world.

Balance the giving and receiving. Put your attention on both sides of the breath. Are the inhalation and exhalation equal in depth and length? Take delight in the balance of giving and receiving. It is a fine equilibrium.

In love relationships, you may feel that you are giving too much and not receiving enough, or you may secretly feel guilty that you are receiving but not giving. You can hurt just as much from having love to give that is not received as you do from wanting to receive love. We all carry around with us an ache or longing, or the memory of an ache or longing, from when love was out of balance. When we allow it, breath will permeate this ache and heal it.

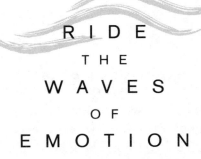

RIDE
THE
WAVES
OF
EMOTION

*B*reath and emotion are completely intertwined. When you breathe freely, you feel freely.

Emotions arise because they have something to teach us, and sometimes they need our full attention. If you want an emotion to disappear, *deal with it*. Then you won't need to revisit it as often.

There are three basic ways to deal with emotion: repression, expression, and assimilation. Each has its time and place. When you **express** something, you speak it or move it and let it flow out into the world. When you **repress** something, you tighten your muscles and hold back expression. When you **assimilate** an emotion, you consciously contain it and learn from it. You track its motion in your inner world. Each of us does all of these all the time—it's part of the craft of being human.

Say you are walking down the street and you see your boyfriend warmly embracing another woman. You are shocked. You want to yell out "Hey!" (expression). In the next breath you find yourself angrily walking faster (repression). You are going to dump him. Then you get closer, and you realize that he's hugging his sister. This all takes place in the matter of several breaths. You laugh to yourself (assimilation). When you get to where they are standing, you can keep the feeling to yourself or share what you just went through. The emotion has been transmuted—it's not shock or jealousy or anger anymore, but rather humor and an affirmation of your bond to this man.

Sometimes the most profound thing to do when you are feeling a strong emotion is to take a deep breath, count to 10, and see what happens. Expression is a wonderful thing, but there are real choices to be made about activating an emotion and putting it into the world, your world, which sometimes means dumping it on others.

Skillful expression of emotion is one of the truly great challenges of being human. When one person expresses herself exceptionally well, as in theater, it can cause catharsis in everyone present. Quiet time is of immense value in managing your emotional life because it gives you time to assimilate the energy of emotions. It is not healthy to just repress an emotion and leave it untended. So, for a moment here and a moment there, even in the midst of a busy day, give yourself some interior space within which to feel.

Exercise Your Ha-Ha
Hee-Hee Ho-Ho Muscles

We can all feel how healthy it is to laugh. Laughter is a great tension releaser. Mirth is a lubricant that lets the gears of life slide smoothly against one another. So take some time now to tap your own funny bone.

Rent a comedy, read the funny pages, or have someone tell you jokes. Go to a comedy club or watch a hit television sitcom. Savor what happens in your belly when you laugh. Get into belly laughter.

After doing that, make "ha-ha," "hee-hee," and "ho-ho" sounds for three breaths each. Explore the different sensations evoked by each sound—they can feel quite different. In my experience, just making these sounds can make you happy.

Experiment with standing, sitting, and lying down, while making these laughing sounds. Yes, that's right, lie down and laugh. If you have a group of people who are reading this book, you can lie in a circle, one person's head on the other's belly, and make laughing sounds.

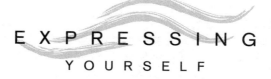

EXPRESSING
YOURSELF

So much of human emotional expression happens on
the outbreath: yelling, growling, crying, laughing, sighing,
ooohing and aahing, and cooing, to name just a few. All of
these are ways of modifying the exhale.

There are situations in life when it is all right to express
emotions without reservation—at the movies (although
some moviegoers might disagree), listening to music, at
sporting events, or with friends. Cheering and booing are
great emotional releases. Thousands of people taking
breath together—often simultaneously—is an awesome experience: great gasps, heavy sighs, exuberant yelps, the
roar of the crowd.

When people give themselves permission to breathe

freely on the exhale and make emotional sounds, they also breathe freely on the inhale. Sporting events, concerts, dances, races, and weddings are all situations in which people breathe in a healthy and free manner. You can learn a lot about breathing from going to these events and letting your breath flow.

As one woman I know puts it, "Anytime I have an emotional release—laughing with people, crying at a movie, telling someone how angry I am about something and growling about it—I find it easier to breathe freely. These things clear me out so that I can feel pleasure in breathing." She continues by pointing out that the release of expression is sometimes quite personal. "Usually, I can't just make the transition from my normal harried life into a breath awareness practice. I just can't. Sometimes, though, at 4 in the morning, I have to. I wake up worrying and then I am forced to breathe in order to calm myself down, and that works."

Recall Times You've Been Emotional

This is a very important exercise and it won't take long. What it will take is a willingness to feel.

Many of us are embarrassed by emotional expressiveness. This embarrassment, as it is ensconced in your breathing muscles, is perhaps your main obstacle to breathing freely. So let's look at ways to deal more fluidly with emotions by focusing on the breath.

Think of times when you have been emotional or have observed others expressing emotions: at movies, plays, weddings, concerts, births, and so forth. What was the impact on your breathing?

Take a moment now, without hurrying, to breathe with each of these feelings for 5 to 10 breaths each:

Eagerness	Laughter
Anger	Fear
Sobbing	Orgasm

Ask friends to name the most moving music and movies they know of and experience these at home. Or, if you are shy about feeling emotions in public, you might want to explore this phenomenon. Go to the theater early, so that you are there as soon as the doors open. Get used to the space so that you feel safe. You can sit there pretending to read a book or newspaper, but just let your eyes rest on the page and pay attention to your breathing. During the movie, give yourself permission to feel fully every emotion that suggests itself—as many as possible. Then stay afterward and breathe with your feelings. There is usually about 10 minutes where you can just sit there undisturbed.

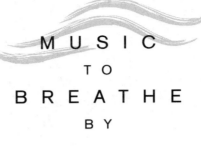

MUSIC
TO
BREATHE
BY

*M*usic expresses feelings that you have but can't articulate. If you pay attention, music shows you how to enter your body, access emotion, and breathe with feeling. This is true of all music, classical and pop. At the same time, breathing with music will help you appreciate it on a deeper level.

Explore the whole range of emotion that the music you love inspires. Consciously acknowledge what that range is, get to know it as you do your taste in food or your choice in clothes. I, for example, love really sad music, such as tragic love songs. I crave to hear them. I find that they resonate in my heart like nothing else. Certain female country-and-western singers embody a quality of feeling—the courage to turn heartache into wine—that I adore. I also appreciate the incredible deep voices of Russian choral singers and the tenor of some Greek Orthodox chants. I have been known to play the latest teen-idol tune followed by Bach. Each expresses emotions I relate to.

If you are feeling very sad, try contradicting the feeling— put on happy music, hopeful music, victory music. In response, you may finally feel free to cry, and let loose with heartrending sobs. Or you might find that the music fills a need and you feel uplifted. Always be prepared for a surprise—you want to be with your feeling as it comes up, not dictate to your heart what it should feel. This is why I recommend cultivating the attitude of an explorer: Be willing to follow where the breath leads.

If you feel hopeless, listen to "Climb Every Mountain" and notice what happens. Rent the movie *Mary Poppins*. There is tremendous therapeutic value in watching musicals. Just remember to breathe consciously with all the emotions the movie engenders in you.

Another mode of exploring your emotions through music is to imagine the soundtrack for what you are feeling in your heart and belly. If you do this over time, you will begin to hear songs—or you may notice that your inner DJ has been playing a melody. There is a tune in your head. When you catch yourself with a song going through your mind, let it be in your body also. Close your eyes and notice what sensations go with the song. Breathe with them. Let the song move your breath to its rhythm, and let your sense of the rich texture of breathing be enhanced by the music. And remember: All music is music to breathe by.

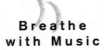

Breathe
with Music

Turn off your telephone ringer and if possible, arrange to not be disturbed. If your living situation doesn't allow you to crank up the music, then get out the headphones.

Lie on the floor with pillows under your head and legs. Turn on your favorite music and listen with your entire body. Let your center of attention be either your heart or your belly and feel the pulsing motion of the breath. Let that be your center of awareness, and listen to the music from there. Keep returning to the rhythm of the breath, drifting back and forth between total involvement in the music and total involvement in the rhythm of the breath. You can learn to appreciate the breath sensation as just another instrument in the band.

Then explore what you can do to satisfy your cravings—the cravings that music awakens—to let the music penetrate your body. Breathe in rhythm with the music. With vocal music, know that these sounds come from an exhale and let your own exhale resonate in sympathy.

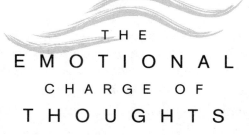

THE
EMOTIONAL
CHARGE OF
THOUGHTS

*F*or months after beginning, women sometimes cry during breath awareness exercises. I believe that most men would cry also, except that they usually stop the exercises rather than let themselves go. At times the tears flow in response to a feeling of grief in the heart, a sensation of words stuck in the throat, or a pang of loneliness. Other times, the tears signal a sense of relief or even joy.

There are many kinds of emotionally charged thoughts: worries about a relationship, worries that you aren't doing enough, or anxiety over some lingering problem. You may feel so much love for someone that you worry about how to show it to them. You might worry about your children:

Can I protect her? Can I provide for him? These are very deep emotions that may surface with a feeling of urgency or dread attached to them. *I must buy that new car because it would be safer for my family,* or *I must fix the fence so the dog can't get out because he might bite someone and they will sue me, then I will lose the house, then I will be homeless, and then how will my grandchildren come and visit me?*

Remember to approach conscious breathing at your own pace, and know that you can regulate your emotions by how much time you spend with the breath. Never forget that the feelings come up because you are allowing them to.

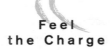

Feel
the Charge

Close your eyes and observe your thoughts as a play of relaxation and tension. Welcome both. You may feel a little bit of inner silence, then a thought or two, then a short movie clip of an action you are planning to do today or did earlier in the day. Then you may think of an activity you should do but don't want to.

Notice the emotional charge that accompanies each thought that comes to mind. This charge may show up as an abstract feeling or something more concrete—a sensation in your throat, your chest, your belly, or somewhere else. It could be an ache—a heartache or an almost-headache. Whatever the sensation, let your awareness rest in it. Doing so will help the emotional tension unfold and release.

DESIRE

*D*esire is a great mystery, and one of life's sacred dynamics. We are going along, living with our usual desires to eat, sleep, talk to friends, and be safe, and then *ouch*, we are struck by another order of desire altogether. We feel a pang in the heart and a yearning for something we do not have—time to go hunting in the woods, or on a pilgrimage to Mecca or Katmandu. We may find ourselves struck by Cupid's arrow and craving a mate. We may long for children, a stable home, a supportive community. The desire could be anything spiritual, emotional, or sensory. We could crave the color turquoise, or long to be seen or heard.

Desire, longing, and yearning are movements toward something. They're the movement of life toward something we feel we need. We are not always aware of why. In the United States and Canada, both very young countries, almost everyone is directly descended from relatively recent immigrants. That means that most of our ancestors were walking around somewhere far from here and one day, bang, they conceived in their hearts the desire to make the risky journey to the New Country.

You do not have to tell anyone your desires when you are in the privacy of your own mind; that is a sacred space, as inviolable as a cathedral. Let the desire come to mind as an image, a feeling, a sound, a smell, or all of these. Then breathe with it. Gradually, you move to being inside the world of the desire, breathing as if the desire were in the act of being fulfilled.

Welcome
Desire Itself

Whenever you practice breath awareness or do anything that leads you into closer contact with your heart and soul, at some point your deeper desires will surface.

Right now, breathe with these concepts and learn to be at home with them.

Desire	Yearning
Longing	Lust

Make sure you can breathe freely with each thought, then move on to others of your own choosing, if you like.

Feel the juice of a desire. Endorse a desire, support it.

Put your awareness into your breath with the intention to clarify the desire. With your breath, give the desire what it needs. Breathe on it like you breathe on a fire to get it started. Feed or nurture it, purify it, separate it or refine it into its essential form, and explore its feeling and ramifications.

Breathe to heal the hurt from desires being unfulfilled. We all have longings in our hearts that are not fulfilled. Breathe with just the right amount of tenderness.

Breathe with the fulfillment of desire.

Desire is movement toward and into another reality. In modern times, people desire to be celebrities; in ancient days, people wanted to be gods.

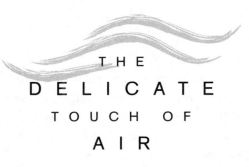

THE
DELICATE
TOUCH OF
AIR

*W*hen you want to be touched, try breath as your masseuse—it has the lightest touch, it will caress you inside and out, and its services are free. Each time you breathe in, the air touches the skin of your nose, then continues to glide along your membranes up behind your face, down your throat, and into the bottom of your lungs by your belly. When you breathe through the mouth, your lips are the first part of you touched by the air, followed by your tongue and the roof of your mouth.

Touch means that there is a boundary—in this case the skin—and something is coming in contact with it. So touch is a relationship you are having. To "be in touch" with yourself means that you are monitoring the touch sensors throughout your body: for temperature, pressure, light touch, hard touch, and the slightest movement of hair follicles. This is a basic activity, mindless really, that simply requires attentiveness. What it gives you in return is a sense of being connected to your environment in a vital way. If you feel isolated or alienated from your community or surroundings, take a walk and pay attention to the parts of your skin that are exposed and the way the breeze touches them.

It's mysterious how breath can seem to flow everywhere in the body at once. If you put your attention on the back of your shoulders, on your legs, on your pelvis—anywhere—and at the same time you are gently aware of your breathing, the sensation will develop that the breath is flowing through that area, massaging it and getting its energies to flow. This has been observed and commented on by the people of ancient India, Tibet, China, Japan, and other places where the life force is explored.

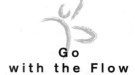

Go
with the Flow

Consider the way your breath flows. Put your hands in front of your nose and move them in and out slightly with the inhale and exhale. Notice the touch of the air on your palms and fingers. Get used to air as something that touches you.

Imagine that the exhaled air pushes your hands out and the inhalation pulls them back in. Notice the coolness of the air as it comes in and the warmth as it flows out. Air is up to 10 degrees warmer on the exhale.

Now move your palms in and out from the area in front of your chest and belly. Notice the sensations of going with the flow.

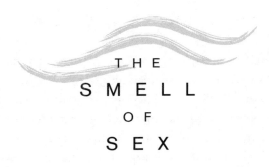

THE
SMELL
OF
SEX

*S*ex is used to sell almost everything. Cars are presented

as sexy. So are men's cologne, women's perfume, clothes,

and shoes.

Smell is a big part of sex. Smell is more intimate than

touch because what we smell goes right into our lungs and

becomes part of our blood almost instantly. Oddly, even

though human beings are deeply influenced by smell at all

times, as a race we are largely unaware of it.

Couples who have been together a long time often

forget those long sessions early on when they were to-

gether with their clothes on, exploring, smelling, tasting,

feeling each other. These activities vitalize a relationship.

Many couples start out well, with lots of sensual bonding, but then they stop for various reasons, take each other for granted, and wind up with more distance between them than they want. Making time to breathe together is very simple. You just have to remember to do it.

Couples who have drifted apart and perhaps are considering separation or divorce may have forgotten how to date each other. Maybe what is appropriate is to act like teenagers and cuddle for a few hours. Just smell and taste each other.

The smell of sex is a blessing because smell as well as touch are vital aspects of bonding with your mate. Reawakening your sense of smell can indeed help rekindle that bond.

Pause in the
Midst of Lovemaking

Sexual arousal is a wave with crests and rests. The joy is in the rhythm. When you let yourself sink deeper into restfulness and relaxation, you are capable of higher highs. Pause in the midst of making love and rest in your breath. Let the smells feed your sexual enjoyment. Really feeling your *yes*, your body's deep response, prepares you to let go more fully.

Taking a moment to sniff your lover may seem strange at first, but go ahead and explore. There are many smells to sex that seem funky at first, especially if you are shy. If you breathe with them, meditate with them, you may find yourself awakening to deep pleasure.

THE
E R O T I C
M A S S A G E   O F
B R E A T H

You may have noticed that sex is best as a full-body experience. It is not just one or two senses—touch and motion—in one part of the body. Sexuality encompasses all the senses—the more the merrier. Ideally, every aspect of the body is involved. We love to see certain things, we love particular smells, there are sounds we want to hear, and there are an infinite number of touches, temperatures, textures, and caresses we want to give and receive.

Sex is not just for reproduction. Lovemaking is an affirmation of the bond between mates, a special time when attention is paid just to each other and no one else. When couples stop finding time for sex, it is usually very hard on the relationship. It is way too easy for couples to get out of sync. Arranging time for sex can be a problem, along with the many other problems we have: finding a partner, keeping a partner, or keeping the love alive and the sparks flying, especially when couples have been together for a while. Again, good lovemaking strengthens the bond between lovers.

If sexual desire is part of your life, breathing has a lot to offer you. Breath awareness activates many senses and prepares them for enjoyment. In order to get ready for sex, you need to slow down; in order to enjoy it, you need to relax enough to let go. Orgasm has much to do with breath—the joy of full and fast breathing. Breathing can help you with all of these.

Many people have surges of sexual desire dozens of times a day, just because they are alive, healthy, and they love life. Each time this happens, the desire does not have to be acted on in any outward way. The desire itself can be savored. Simply breathe with it for a minute and let it electrify you. Sexual energy, when cherished, circulates to every sensory pathway until even looking at a tree in the afternoon sun is an erotic experience. When sexual desire is appreciated in this way, it adds a great deal of zest to life.

In interviewing people over the years, one thing comes across: Almost no one gets enough massage or enough simple, loving caresses. I interviewed a massage therapist who lives in Big Sur, California, and for 30 years has taught massage in an astoundingly beautiful location on a cliff overlooking the Pacific Ocean. She sighed when I asked her if she receives enough touch. She told me she went to massage school partly in order to get touched, but the kind of caress she craves is so subtle that it requires an infinite patience few men, even men in her profession, can give. I think that what she craves is the kind of touch that only breath can give.

Years ago I got up one morning and wrote in my journal, "Meditation is for passions so deep that they cannot be fulfilled by ordinary life experience." I think of breath massage as being this way also—it is for the ways we crave to be touched that no human hand can satisfy.

Our animals love to be touched and stroked, but we ourselves do not get our fair share. Women in particular have a hankering for leisurely, delicate stroking. Everyone has different cravings for touch: fast, slow, here, there.

Desire is a mystery to be explored. If you explore and give yourself this luxury, you will be filled up with it. You will be able to give it to your lover and thus will be more likely to receive it. The cycle has to start somewhere.

Explore Erotic Breath

If you like, take a shower or bath and light a candle, just as you would for a romantic evening. Have a playful, exploratory attitude. Sometimes you have to catch yourself as you are, so if you want to, you can do this exercise outside in nature, in your car while parked somewhere, or at your desk if you have to. If you want to do it covertly, just pretend that you are meditating.

If there's a particular scent that you like or find erotic (either a woman's or a man's scent), place it on the inside of one wrist or at the place where your thumb and forefinger come together. Inhale this scent for a dozen breaths, feeling what happens all over your body as you do so. Inhale through your nose and exhale through your mouth.

With your mouth slightly open, breathe in and notice the

tender touch of the air as it flows over those sensitive nerve endings in your lips. (You may want to use lip moisturizer if they get dry.) Continue in this way with all attention on your lips.

Play with varying the shape of your lips. You will notice the sensations change with each almost imperceptible shift in the way you shape your lips.

Then let your attention move to the top of your tongue, the roof of your mouth, and the empty space between them. Rest your attention on the stimulation your tongue and roof are receiving.

Next become aware of the back of your throat and the way it receives the air. Notice how the air is warmer and moister as it glides up and out than when it goes down.

Then become aware of the breath expanding your chest slightly, pushing your breasts outward. This is a very subtle sensation. If you want to amplify it, you could wear something silky.

Rest your attention in your belly, feeling it rising and falling, expanding and contracting.

Become aware of your pelvis and of the very tiny sensations that are evoked by the motion of your belly just above it. Usually, we do not pay attention to breath in the lower torso. When you first start noticing, it may be like walking into a dark theater. You can't see where the seats are. Over several minutes, your senses will adapt and you will start to perceive the rocking motion of breath as it flows. As you pay attention, the sensations will tend to get stronger there.

Be aware of the whole flow of breath downward, from your throat to your chest to your belly on down. Imagine that the breath touches your genital area before turning back and going upward.

Then let your awareness be global again. Be aware of your skin all over, and luxuriate in the feeling of being contained within your skin and your aura. You may have a soft tingling sensation in your skin, or the sense of being inside an invisible blanket.

Sit there for a while, resting in the delicious feelings.

Share
a Breath

With a partner, become aware of the palms of both of your hands. Rub them together or breathe on them—or breathe on each other's palms to awaken them.

Then touch each other lightly, anywhere.

As you touch your partner somewhere with your palm, imagine that you are sending your breath into him, blessing him and letting him know on a very deep level how much you love him. Cherish the fact that he exists here, in a human body.

Receive your lover's touch so that you feel touched inside by his love. As you inhale, allow yourself to take in his essence, his touch, as you take in the air.

Now feel your lover's breath. Ask him to breathe on your chest, your lower back, between your shoulder blades—anywhere. Use your imagination. While he does, breathe with him. First explore pulse breath, when you inhale and exhale at the same time as your partner. Then try counterpoint breath, where you breathe in while he breathes out, and vice versa. Continue to enjoy the erotic experience of taking breaths together.

After sharing breath in this way for a while, you might like to try the Spine-Tingling Breath. Ask your partner to touch you very lightly along your spine, from your tailbone to your neck. Have him slowly run his fingers up, touching lightly. Then have him use just the breath—touching your skin with his breath, up and down your spine, with great leisure.

Do this with each other and then sit or lie down and meditate with the breath.

One of the things you can learn from this exercise is just how electrifying breath can be. Memorize the feeling and let it permeate your entire body. Someone once told me that the feeling made them want to jump out of their skin. It is just that feeling you want to cultivate—but don't jump out of your skin. Instead, ride the electricity in the other direction and it will pleasure your nerve endings in ways of which you never dreamed.

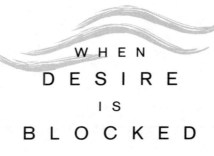

WHEN DESIRE IS BLOCKED

*W*hen a desire is frustrated, other emotions arise: frustration, anger, fear, anxiety, depression. Losing an object of desire leads to grief. What frustrations and disappointments have you known? What happens to your breathing now when you recall them?

Anger is nature's bulldozer. It gives you extra oomph when a desire is thwarted. It gets a bad rap, deservedly, because it can be so destructive, but in essence anger is pro-life. The movement of anger is outward, explosive. The movement is to get something out, to push through or push someone or something away.

When you are angry, you may want to take a really full

breath, to huff and puff and blow the house down, to inflate your whole aura. Anger is fire, anger is power. Anger can grant you the gift of alertness, even if you can't act on it.

Breathe with Anger

To begin, access the even rhythm of your breath for 1 to 2 minutes. That is your security and your anchor, which makes it safe to dive into the wildness of anger. When things get too intense, just return to the steady, full circulation of air through your lungs.

Now think of something that makes you angry, and breathe with it. It could be something that is affecting you presently, or it could be a memory from your past. Think about how much it hurt you or something you value, and savor the feeling of wanting to yell about it, hit something, or destroy the situation that is hurting you. Give your anger full room to teach you about itself.

Any of these can help you liberate the energy behind your anger:

- Express yourself in movement. Open your mouth and show your teeth as you pant. Pump your breath by working your diaphragm, to liberate the energy in your solar plexus. You might try the Jazz Your Breath exercise on page 107.

- Slowly get bigger. Take slow, full, deliberate breaths. Create more inner space for the anger to fill. Your diaphragm, ribs, and belly can be filled with your fire. Your whole space is charged. Your boundaries are strong. *Nobody can mess with me!*

➤ Do pushing-away movements. Breathe out to expurgate the unwanted energies or sensations. Growl, snort, and exhale fully and forcefully. Stomp your feet. Pump your arms up and down. Punch the air. Hit a pillow. Yell out "No no no!" Breathe fast. Strike. These are the movements of anger, and doing them will help you release it from being stuck in your body.

➤ People like to exercise when they are angry. This is extremely healthy and instinctively wise. Even if you know how to meditate, check out exercising hard when you get angry. You are channeling the power of the anger to move your muscles. Your breath is pumping life, so the energy of anger does not get bottled up.

Give yourself over to the energy of the anger without acting out on others. Then pause and feel the clarity of the energy running through you. This is a victory, that you can feel your anger without having to either block it, repress it, or act it out.

In that clarity, decide what needs to be done in the outer world, ethically.

Match Your Anger

Sometimes to release anger you may want to match it first. Matching your anger means that you completely honor and acknowledge it within yourself. You feel it but do not act on it in any way, and then you provide your own healing by treating yourself well. It's true that sometimes living well really is the best revenge.

To match your anger, breathe fast—even faster than you would when panting with anger. Sit and pump the air rapidly in and out of your belly for 1 to 3 minutes. That is a way of safely acknowledging the anger. Instead of thinking of any images or memories, focus purely on your bodily sensations. Breathing rapidly will give you lots of sensations to note.

Now shift to the soothing phase. You might want to lie down for this. Take long, deep breaths and impose an even rhythm on your breathing. This will take a minute or so.

Then put your attention on letting your breath wash through your entire body from your head to your toes. Feel the breath gently clearing the anger out of your body with its cool, refreshing flow.

On the exhale, feel the anger being released from your body. As you inhale, feel fresh new energy entering your body.

Toward the end of this exercise, put your hands on your heart and breathe in soothing energy. Feel yourself coming into balance. As the breath streams through your whole body, the anger turns into sensations of increased circulation and a pleasurable sense of your own power.

Reflect on the saying "This too shall pass" and become poised, awaiting further developments.

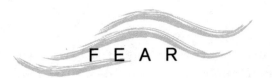

FEAR

*C*heck in with your breathing. Is it free and easy? If not, why not? Are you hiding from something? Engage the fear. Anchor yourself in your breath, get comfortable and safe in your breath, then let your fear unfold itself completely.

The movement of fear is that of moving away from a threat, or sometimes becoming still and invisible like a hunted animal. Your body's response is the same whether you are in physical danger or you imagine an abstract situation and feel threatened on some level. While you can usually escape an actual situation, it's hard to get away when the threat is something you imagine. If you can neither fight nor flee, you become paralyzed. Recover the ability for contact and withdrawal.

Fear in modern people often results in paralysis. Animals, when they can, just run away. Human beings often find themselves in situations where they can't hit someone and they can't run away either. This is a good thing in the larger picture, but it is difficult for the body to figure out how to handle, and it can create an instinctive stalemate. Another set of instincts kicks in—to hide. Restricting the breathing, making it shallow, and controlling the belly is a natural response if you are a deer hiding from a mountain lion. If you are hiding, you try to make yourself small, invisible, and quiet. If your life is in danger from a tiger lurking on the cliff above you, then it is appropriate to breathe shallowly. Maybe he won't hear you. Maybe he won't smell your breath.

When you take time to be with yourself and relax into the breath, you may find that your body is filled with fear. You may realize you have been in a situation in which your fear response is always activated. Maybe someone new at work is threatening to take your job. You can't run away, but you're not sure how to respond. If you find that your body has a sense of being paralyzed by fear, you might want to match the fear. You can do that with a sense of playing.

Match
Your Fear

Breathe as quietly as you can for about a minute, as if you were hiding from some imminent danger. You could even physically cower and shrink yourself down. Access the feeling of fleeing and let yourself know that you can run away if you really need to.

Now counter your fear. Access the feeling of your own power. Engage the muscles in your legs and your arms, as if you were readying yourself to pounce.

Then let go of this skit and focus on the movement and flow of breath. Notice that here and now you can breathe freely. Gradually, you will find the breath easing out of fear into fullness and comfort. Breathe and let the fear be washed out of your body.

Fear is a real problem in modern society. Many people I meet live in totally inappropriate fear. Statistically, people who live in a city in the modern Western world are safer than anyone who has ever lived that we have knowledge of. The average life span is longer than ever, well over the age of 60. Yet people walk around quivering in fear and are afraid to walk down the street because of violence they hear about and see on television.

Whenever you take the time to breathe consciously, fear will be washed out of your body and you will be that much more able to face the world and live in reality as it is, not as your fears imagine it to be.

SORROW

Sorrow is the feeling we have when we need to let go of something we have cherished. Sorrow comes from loss, and it is an appropriate response. The sensations inspired by sorrow can vary from an emptying out to a sinking feeling. It is a small death that, if you let it, gives your body and mind a chance to be reborn to a fresh start in life. In experiencing sorrow, your heart becomes tender and you open yourself to the smallest gifts that life presents. If you let yourself really breathe in the feeling, you'll discover a poignancy, an almost unbearable sweet sorrow to life. This gives rise, in turn, to a compassion born of passion.

Oftentimes in life we are exposed to devastating pain. Sometimes it is from the death of a loved one. Sometimes it is from abuse or betrayal. Sometimes there is loss of other kinds—a dream dies, we have to move and we lose our community, or a relationship changes into a form we do not like. Sometimes several of these losses happen simultaneously or in the same year, and it is as if life as we know it is gone, and we are in darkness.

In other words, there are times when it is hard to breathe, when each breath is painful because it massages the heart and your heart hurts.

Sink into Sorrow

Even a little bit of breath awareness can help you deal with this difficult emotion called sorrow. Realize that every exhalation is a loss, a giving up, an emptying out. When you breathe out, you sink down, and if you do not fear this sinking, it will put you on the path to healing. The sinking down is the death that can lead to resurrection. So how best to breathe with sorrow? Match it.

- Sigh
- Exhale loudly
- Empty yourself and wait
- Wail

People who are grieving sometimes say things such as, "I feel like sinking into the ground." One exploration you could do is to stand and then literally sink with sorrow. Let your shoulders slump, hang your head, then sink down and collapse. Lie on the ground and breathe. Let your spirit sink into the ground, into the Earth. Sink into sorrow with the exhale. Let yourself collapse and melt.

Now inhale and feel the tender gift of breath coming in and healing your heart.

Hold your heart with the breath. Rock forward and back and hum soothingly to yourself.

If all else fails, many people find that the most essential emotional release, the key action that grants access to the others, is crying. Being able to let go and sob over life's hurts is a direct way to free up the breathing muscles because they are the very same muscles we use to hold back our tears and our anger.

If you like, let it all out.

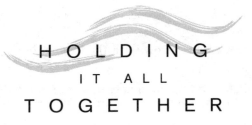

HOLDING
IT ALL
TOGETHER

You may be distressed, exhausted, or feel like crying or giving up, but most of the time, you still manage to hold it all together. Fear is a motivating factor: If you fall apart you will let down loved ones, or others will see you as vulnerable and be tempted to take advantage. What may happen, though, is that you get stuck just holding on and forget how to truly let go. You may think you are being responsible, but if you are not getting enough rest and relaxation, your performance will surely degrade.

When we fall asleep, we fall apart in a way that benefits both body and mind. You can consciously build times to fall apart into your daily waking life as well. Falling apart is psychologically and emotionally breathing out. At the end of an exhale, for example, you do not know if you will ever breathe in again. Truly, breathing is an act of trust.

When you are anxious or under pressure, your solar plexus tightens and becomes like a fist. When you relax that fist, everything else lets go. You may feel fear that you are stumbling and might fall behind. But you never know what is on the other side of tightness—sometimes it is ecstasy.

I find it wise that people all over the world go to karaoke bars in the evening and cut loose. Learn to not be afraid of your spontaneity. Holding in your emotions all the time can lead to a chronic sense that what is inside of you is harmful somehow, and that to protect others or yourself you have to keep it in check. This is a shame.

The knowledge of how to let go is there in your body, and the breath will gladly show you how. If you pay attention, you will see that when you are tired, you naturally let go as you exhale and your grip on the world relaxes for a few seconds.

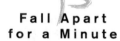

Fall Apart
for a Minute

Here is an exercise you can practice anytime you have a minute—and there is always a minute here or there in a day.

You can safely let yourself fall apart for a brief period. The world will carry on without you. To prove this to yourself, explore what would happen if you didn't hold it all together. Do this in the safety of your own body.

Close your eyes for 60 seconds and breathe out with a sigh. As you do so, release control of your breath, your belly, and your armor. Fall into the exhale. Muscles all over your body will begin to relax. Let the inbreath happen of its own accord, then exhale again with a sigh. Every 5 seconds you are letting go, and every 5 seconds you are being revived by the inbreath.

You can practice anything for 5 seconds, even if it is against your nature. Even if you think of yourself as a failure at relaxation, you actually are good at it in 5-second increments. Just keep coming back to it 5 seconds at a time. Pulse, the world dissolves; pulse, it reappears. Your nervous system is used to this 4- to 5-second pulsation of the breath, so that is all you have to tolerate—a few seconds at a time.

When you are exhaling, after a moment you may feel like a puddle, completely vulnerable. Or you may feel like nothing and nobody—worthless. You may feel guilty for resting. These are itty-bitty sensations, nothing worth exerting yourself to block out. You do not have to deal with these sensations; simply tolerate them being there and do not interfere. The breath will support you and carry you. It will let you sink and relax, and then it will lift you up so you can go on.

Again, close your eyes and let the world fall apart, this time for 3 minutes. At the end of that time, slowly open your eyes and permit yourself to be resurrected. Notice how relieved you are when you breathe out.

People in recovery like to say that they are taking things one day at a time. But sometimes a day is too big to handle. If you can take things one breath at a time, you can work your recovery from chronic tension to relaxation.

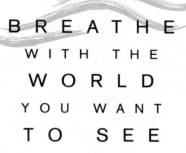

BREATHE
WITH THE
WORLD
YOU WANT
TO SEE

*S*ome people just know, innately, that they are God's

worker bees. They don't question their desires or motiva-

tion. Such people make themselves happy, and because

they do, they radiate an energy I enjoy.

I once talked with an industrious businessman in his

early thirties who lived in a state of vital interest in his

work and in the world. I was asking him about his plans

for the future. As we were walking along, I saw him do an

unconscious breath technique. He looked at the horizon,

his pupils expanded slightly, he took a moderately strong

breath, and then he refocused. The whole thing took

5 to 7 seconds, I would guess. Then he turned back to me, not having missed a beat in the conversation.

I asked him what he had just been thinking. He was surprised and didn't know how to answer. But after a bit of questioning, he said that he had been visualizing the kind of house he was planning to buy, which would be paid for by the sale of one of his businesses. He knew the area and the view he wanted, and in his imagination he was standing in the house, enjoying the light, and taking a breath.

Watching him, I realized what a perfect technique this is for him. It keeps him energized and it relates his working life to nest building, which keeps him breathing easily. He is not waiting until he physically steps into his new home to breathe with such enthusiasm; rather, visualizing the goal he is working toward gives him the energy to get there. This is part of his automatic, unconscious healthiness. Every half-hour or so he thinks of something like this that he loves, and he shares a breath with it. He draws strength from it. He sips from life's elixir in this way. I have no doubt that when he has children he will continue with the same strategy—keeping what he loves in his heart and breathing with it regularly.

Also, his execution of it is wonderful. Since the technique is unconscious and natural, it is not tedious. He sees his vision, takes a breath with it, and moves on.

As you absorb the ideas and the exercises in this book, your body and mind will take what is appropriate for you, subtly improving your life skills, with some of the practices becoming a working part of your unconscious. Ideally, you won't even know you are practicing anything. This doesn't mean that you have become unconscious of breathing, as you were before, but that the enjoyment of breath taking has become a seamless part of your life.

Breathe
with the Sun

Have you ever wondered where oxygen comes from? Astrophysicists theorize that large stars, somewhat larger than our sun, generate vast amounts of oxygen in the mature part of their life cycles and then explode and breathe it out into space. So when you turn your attention to the stars, you can thank them for providing the oxygen you are breathing.

When we are with the breath on a sunny day, it sometimes seems as if we metabolize sunlight directly—the sun charges the air with some life-giving quality that we absorb when we inhale. While we breathe with the light, our skin and eyes seem to feed on the luminosity. Even when we come inside, the glow that we feel lingers.

Go outside and take a walk in the sunlight. What time of day provides your favorite luster—dawn, sunset, late afternoon, or high noon? Arrange to be in the light at that time and breathe with it. Savor the radiance of the sun, the touch of the light on your skin, and the flow of your breath as it enters your body and circulates inside you. Imagine the light gently diffusing throughout your entire system.

Allow yourself the space and the breath to realize your love for light. Feed on the light as you inhale; feel the warm energy coming into your lungs and reviving you. Rest in the light. Be massaged and soothed and cleansed by the light. Make love to light as you breathe. Light is food for the eyes and food for the brain. If possible, expose your entire body to the sun for 20 minutes in a safe place, resting and breathing in the light. You can also use visualization, sitting inside but conjuring up the memory of being outdoors in the sun.

Breathe
with the Wind

There is one body of air surrounding this planet, and you are breathing it. It circulates freely, and as it flows it creates movement in the trees, waves on the water, tornadoes and dust devils on the plains. It carries the clouds that bring rain. As you breathe, you are participating in this planetary dance.

Go outside where you can see the movement of leaves, branches, clouds, or ripples and waves on water. There may be a flag blowing in the breeze, or a plastic bag bouncing in an eddy. If you can't be outside right now, visualize one or more of these images. But as soon as you can, go out into nature and breathe with the wind.

Breathe
with the Colors

We can have cravings for color just as we can crave specific touches, tastes, or sounds. Breathe with the colors and infuse yourself with light; after all, what is color but light?

Humans are capable of discerning seemingly countless hues, each of which elicits a different effect or feeling. The color you crave may exist in nature—think of exotic birds, butterfly wings, tropical fish, fresh fruit, and wildflowers—or you may rely on your imagination to conjure the perfect shade. There may be a range of colors you love, the way the horizon changes hues moment by moment at sunset, with reds transitioning into blues and violets and sometimes even greens.

Make yourself comfortable anywhere and think of a color you love. You could be outdoors in nature, or you could look at colorful photographs, fabric, or paintings. Go to a museum or gallery and breathe with art you love. If it's erotic art, breathe with the different colors and shapes of flesh, letting them permeate your breath and your body. Then close your eyes and rest, relishing the aftereffects.

Visualize your own breath as color. You breathe in the color, it is absorbed by your lungs, and it is distributed through your body and metabolized by your cells. Then breathe out that same color, or perhaps one a little brighter. You have absorbed some of the color, and it flows through your body.

Breathing with utter black can be especially refreshing, although technically black indicates the absence of color. (White is all of the colors combined.) Arrange to be in total blackness for 5 minutes or more, and be aware of your breathing. You can get this effect by putting on a blindfold or by lying down and putting a towel over your eyes.

If you do this exercise on different days, you may discover that you crave different colors to satisfy different instinctive needs: soothing, warmth, healing, peace, energy. Or you may just plain love the colors.

Breathe with the Vastness

Lie on your back gazing up at the heavens, in a wide-open place under a cloudless sky; lie beneath the night sky with the stars overhead; or stand on a mountaintop or on the roof of a building and look at the horizon, at the vista. Let your awareness encompass the vastness, and then let your attention rest in your belly. Realize that the air you are breathing came from out there—the horizon, the distant stars. Alternate between being in your belly and being with the vastness. Feel the breath flowing deep into your belly, then release it to flow far away.

Have your eyes wide open, taking in the vastness. Send your attention out over the distance. Then close your eyes and continue to feel this vastness as you breathe. On the inhalation, breathe the universe into yourself. Remind yourself that the stars breathe out oxygen, and some ancient star breathed out the very oxygen you are breathing in now. On the exhalation, breathe out as if you are giving back to the stars the material to form new planets.

Another thing you can do is rent the movie *Contact*, starring the actress Jodie Foster. Watch the first 5 minutes several times: A fantastic view of the universe zooms out from a spot on Earth. The imagery is based on photographs from the Hubble telescope, radio astronomy, and computer modeling.

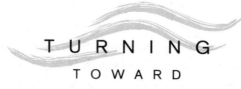

TURNING
TOWARD

*W*hen a human being turns toward the ultimate source of energy in the universe, this is called prayer (unless you are a scientist—then it is called astrophysics).

This turning-toward motion is built into living things. In biology it is called tropism—all living beings turn toward their source of sustenance. There is hydrotropism, when plants grow toward water, and heliotropism, when living things turn toward light. In beings that are conscious, such as humans and possibly animals (pets), this turning toward can manifest itself as a love relationship.

Tropism-related images—God as light and the Holy Spirit as living water—appear in prayers: "He leadeth me by the still waters" or "The Lord is my Light." We can see that religion is something that comes from deep within and relates our most personal needs to the infinite.

The Psalms of David, beloved of Jews, Christians, and Muslims (Muhammad taught that there are four inspired books: the Torah of Moses, the Psalms of David, the Gospel of Jesus Christ, and the Koran), are a great and versatile source of such imagery, and a veritable map of the human heart. Throughout the 150 or so Psalms, a vast array of predicaments, dilemmas, conundrums, and perplexities are described, and a mosaic of almost every human emotion is set forth.

Adoration, gratitude:
". . . delight is in the law of the Lord . . ."
Psalm 1

Protection:
". . . thou, O Lord, art a shield for me . . ."
Psalm 3

Bonding:
"O Lord my God, in thee do I put my trust . . ."
Psalm 7

Rest:
". . . he leadeth me beside the still waters.
He restoreth my soul . . ."
Psalm 23

Revenge:
"Let them all be confounded . . ."
Psalm 129

Pray for what you feel you need while focusing on receiving the inbreath. Notice that you are actually taking a substance, the substance of Spirit, into your body right now. This helps create the feeling of receiving what the prayer is referring to. In this way, breath awareness complements the experience of prayer.

Breathe with the
Rhythm of a Prayer

When you talk to the universe, what do you say? *Help me! Heal me. Give me strength. Let me rest. Please protect me.* These are all core concerns of prayer. What do you wish for others? Peace, harmony, love, infinite joy? Whatever your pleasure, praying for it turns your attention toward that need, and your whole being becomes alerted to the possibility of receiving that quality from life.

The next step is breathing with your prayer. This requires a sense of leisure, play, exploration, curiosity, and a trust of the silence between words.

There is no law that says you must hurry up and finish a prayer within 15 seconds. I encourage you to take your time. Explore the spirit of the prayer, breathe with it, drink from its well. You may become aware of the continuous flow of breath carrying the meaning of the prayer, massaging you with the vibrational tone of the prayer. The breath turnings are pause points where you can dwell and feel the impact of the prayer. With each outbreath, give the breath to God. Give the gratitude to God. With each inbreath, receive from God the answer to the prayer. Exhale and surrender to your yearning. Inhale and receive the blessing into your needy cells. Take the prayer deep into your body and your soul and rest in it.

Let my sexual energies be in the
service of my soul evolution.

Let my gut instincts serve the integration of my life.

Let my heart energies encompass
and bless all those I love.

Let my speech articulate the truth.

Let my insight be clear.

May I know oneness of soul and spirit.

Whispering a prayer, you can feel it being carried out on your breath, an offering on the altar of the universe. The song of your prayer is as much a part of the music of the world as are the songs of whales and wolves, birds and crickets. Also explore walking very slowly with the rhythm of the breath and the rhythm of the prayer setting your pace.

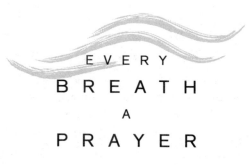

EVERY
BREATH
A
PRAYER

Let everything that hath breath praise the Lord.

—PSALM 150

*B*reath is sacred. Every breath you breathe is a breath with God. The intimacy of prayer and breath is embodied in the word "spirit," as in the Holy Spirit. As we take a small amount of this air into our bodies and embrace it within ourselves, the spirit becomes part of us.

You do not have to imagine that you are in contact with God because you are already experiencing that contact in a direct way through your senses. As one of my favorite sutras puts it, "Every breath you breathe is an unconscious prayer. To breathe in and breathe out is an act of worship to the Lord of Life."

Prayer is a turning toward that which gives us life, sustains us, and renews us. When we say "Give us this day our daily bread," we are acknowledging God as the ultimate source of food. When we turn in gratitude toward God for the next breath, it is the same idea, for air is a kind of food. Gratitude for each breath is the highest teaching that there is in meditation, and also the simplest practice.

Bask in Gratitude
for Each Breath

Right now, sit back and for a moment be grateful for your breath. Simply bask in gratitude to be alive and that each breath is sustaining your life. Think of the greatest experience you have ever had, the most love or the most fun you have ever had, and be grateful to the breath. You might say to yourself out loud, "I give thanks for this breath." Then breathe out and be silent, savoring the release of the old air. If you don't feel comfortable saying anything aloud, simply think of the world and all its oceans and forests, which are continually generating oxygen, and be grateful for those vast expanses as you breathe. Or, if you prefer, simply give thanks directly to God, whatever your concept of Him (or Her) is.

This is a wonderful practice to do every day for at least a minute. Try it. The gratitude will permeate your body and your life, like when you add a drop of flavoring or a smidgen of spice to food. Then you can easily return to this simple attitude again and again as you go about your day.

Become
a Living Soul

Genesis 2:7 reads, "And the Lord God formed man of the dust of the ground, and breathed into his nostrils the breath of life; and man became a living soul."

You can take this verse to be in the present tense and use it as a breathing meditation: *God is breathing into my nostrils the breath of life, and I am a living soul.* By paying attention to the inbreath through the nostrils, you can be there to meet the inflowing spirit. In practice, this means only a tiny shift of awareness—you are appreciating the inbreath as a gift of divinity. I find this an extremely exciting practice that is endlessly interesting.

You can do this for one breath at the beginning of the day, or you can make a walking meditation of it and dwell with the quote from Genesis as you go about your business. If you want to meditate more formally with this scripture, sit comfortably somewhere you feel safe—in your church, or in your favorite spot in your house or garden. If feasible, arrange to be undisturbed. With your eyes open, look around at the world for a minute or two, simply noting the distance of each thing from you: There is a wall, here is a tree, and over there is a chair. While you look about, become aware of the empty space between you and the items—there is a boundary of air around you. Then, when you feel like it, close your eyes.

If you feel it is appropriate, ask God or the Holy Spirit to guide you in meditation.

Turn your awareness toward your nostrils and gently pervade that whole area of your nose with your attention. Become awake in the nose, at the doorway through which the breath of life flows, as if you were greeting someone at the door of your home. Welcome the air flowing in for a minute and get used to how your rhythm feels today. Then, with a great amount of leisure, begin to think the phrase, *God is breathing into my nostrils the breath of life*. If you want to vary that thought in any way, or condense it, go ahead. It is the thought that counts, not the exact phrasing.

Think the phrase every minute or so. There will be a particular rhythm you find charming and restful, so go with that. Hear the words in your mind—*God is breathing into my nostrils the breath of life*—and then rest in your breath and simply appreciate what a marvelous feeling this is. Continue to enjoy the sensations of breath. After a dozen or so breaths, think the phrase again.

Lift Your Hands to Heaven

Lift your hands slowly above your head and hold them there comfortably. Note the uplifting feeling. Explore the difference in feeling when you have your palms facing each other and then facing forward. Notice the energy in the space above your head. Then rest your hands in your lap and savor the sensations.

Breathe fairly rapidly for about a minute, then repeat. Raise your hands again for about 30 seconds, then rest them in your lap again.

Bless your body. Bless every part of your body. Give thanks for the life-giving breath. Breath permeates even the areas of you that you don't like, that you want to change. The breath is everywhere.

On the outgoing breath, bless all those you love. On the incoming breath, receive love from Christ, God, Allah, Ishwara.

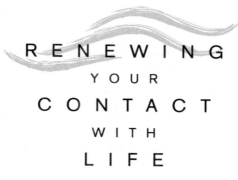

RENEWING
YOUR
CONTACT
WITH
LIFE

*W*hen you begin to breathe more enthusiastically, life

may bite back. You may discover that people were used to

you being quieter, more repressed. You may discover that

your musculature is used to your keeping a low profile and

not taking much from or giving much to life. So go at your

own pace and get help if you need to. There are breath

teachers everywhere: your nearest dance teacher, rabbi,

priest, imam, therapist, physical therapist, voice teacher,

chef, wine taster, choir leader, swimming coach. Each one

knows about an aspect of breath that the others have not

explored.

As you extend and refine your sensory perception, it affects all domains of your life. When your sense of color and shape is awakened because you have studied photography or painting, you see everything in an enriched way. If you amplify your kinesthesia through dance or massage, the increased body awareness carries over into walking, making love, and even sleeping.

As you breathe more freely, you will feel your own life more intensely and you will discover lots of new things about yourself and the world. Tiny perceptions will strike you as novel. You will have changed, however slightly, your baseline of perception.

Most of what you will encounter are tiny shifts in your sensual experience of the world in the direction of becoming less numb. And the feeling is one of surprise more than anything because you *do* know all your senses—you have just forgotten about them. People commonly forget to enjoy their senses for 10 to 20 years at a time, and then when they come to their senses again it is as if no time has passed. It's a bit like seeing an old friend.

The purpose of this book has been to inspire you to cultivate your sensory awareness of breathing and thereby point you toward an enriched sense of life in general.

The secret of breath taking is this: Don't resist the motion of life.

GRATITUDE

Explorations

In developing this book, I have been blessed to be surrounded and entertained by an enchanted circle of friends who are also exploring the breath in its many dimensions. Foremost among these is Camille Maurine, my wife, who took time away from dancing to toss off many great ideas and useful corrections as she strode through the papers I left all over the living room floor. For decades, Camille has been exploring breath as it relates to movement meditation and theater. She is also a great attack-ninja editor—anything that makes her brow furrow gets tossed. Her work is called *kinAesthetics*, and you can find out more about it by visiting www.camillemaurine.com. Read *Meditation Secrets for Women* by Camille Maurine and Lorin Roche (HarperSanFrancisco, 2001).

For many years, Camille studied and taught Continuum, a courageous and openhearted movement-meditation form developed by Emilie Conrad. During the writing of this book, Emilie graciously gave her time in many hilarious, free-ranging discussions about breath. Since Emilie and I both get up at outrageous hours to write—often 3:00 or 4:00 A.M.—by 10 in the morning we are almost drunk on the sheer zaniness of attempting to describe meditative experience in words. So when we talk in the late morning, it's as if we're in a bar in the wee hours, after a bottle of wine each. For information about Continum workshops, visit www.continuummovement.com or call (310) 453-4402.

Michael Batliner, my swimming buddy, spent many hours going over the ideas in this book with me as we cruised through the chilly but soul-warming waters of Malibu. In particular, I am grateful for the parts of the conversation that occurred while we were out in the ocean, treading water and talking about some nuance of the inhalation. Michael has been studying and teaching Middendorf Breathwork, an extremely refined set of methods for engaging with the living breath. For more information, contact The Middendorf Breath Institute, 435 Vermont Street, San Francisco, CA 94107, or call them at (415) 255-2174.

Marshall Ho, my tai chi teacher from 1968 onward, gave me the original inspiration for much of what is in this book. Marshall shared himself with an intense generosity and showed us the delight behind the graceful motions of tai chi. I consider tai chi to be one of the Great Things and a wonderful gift that the Chinese have given the world. There are classes everywhere, and you can learn a lot from videos as well.

Ed Maupin gave me many incredible bodywork sessions in the late 1960s at the Esalen Institute, which opened up my breathing and my entire body to the flow of vitality. Ed combined deep-tissue Rolfing (Structural Integration) with movement exploration, sensory awareness, and imagery.

Thanks also to Dorothy Nolte, a Rolfer and movement awareness teacher, who worked with me very deeply for an entire year in 1969–1970, and was instrumental in my awakening into the marvels of breath.

⬤

Thanks to my father, Richard Roche, and my mother, Myra, for taking me out into the ocean almost from my first breath. To get a sense of the magical world of wind, waves, and sand, see the photographic essay *Surfing San Onofre to Point Dume, 1936–1942* (Chronicle Books, 1998) by family friend Don James.